# Challenging cancer

*Challenging Cancer* shows people with cancer how they can stop feeling like victims and regain control of their lives. Dr Nira Kfir, a psychotherapist specialising in crisis intervention, and Dr Maurice Slevin, a cancer physician, describe how cancer patients can use the crisis that cancer brings about rather than be used by it.

The book provides a unique opportunity to share the experiences of cancer patients and to learn from their insights. Group discussions at cancer workshops are reported verbatim, revealing patients' strategies for coping with the crisis in their lives and showing how they become actively involved rather than allowing things to happen to them. The book also tells the remarkable story of the late Vicky Clement Jones, well known as the founder of BACUP, the British Association of Cancer United Patients. The exceptional process of Vicky's treatment, medical as well as psychological, transformed her from a highly scientific doctor to a social reformer who achieved, through her illness, the creation of a concept and an organisation.

*Challenging Cancer* will be of enormous help to all cancer patients, their families and friends; and to doctors, nurses and social workers.

**Nira Kfir** is a psychotherapist and the Director of the Maagalim Psychotherapy Institute in Tel Aviv. She is the author of *Crisis Intervention Verbatim* (New York: Hemisphere, 1988). **Maurice Slevin** is a consultant cancer physician at St Bartholomew's and Homerton Hospitals in London. He is Chairman of BACUP (British Association of Cancer United Patients).

# Challenging cancer

## From chaos to control

Nira Kfir and Maurice Slevin

Foreword by Anthony Clare

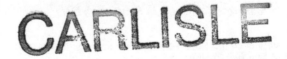

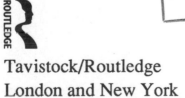
Tavistock/Routledge
London and New York

First published in 1991
by Routledge
11 New Fetter Lane, London EC4P 4EE

Simultaneously published in the USA and Canada
by Routledge
a division of Routledge, Chapman and Hall Inc.
29 West 35th Street, New York, NY 10001

Reprinted 1992

Typeset by LaserScript Ltd, Mitcham, Surrey
Printed and bound in Great Britain by
Mackays of Chatham PLC, Chatham, Kent

*British Library Cataloguing in Publication Data*

Kfir, Nira
    Challenging cancer.
    1. Humans. Cancer.
    I. Title II. Slevin, Maurice
    616.99406

*Library of Congress Cataloging in Publication Data*

Kfir, Nira
    Challenging cancer: from chaos to control/Nira Kfir
        and Maurice Slevin.
    p. cm.
    Includes index.
    1. Cancer – Psychological aspects. 2. Cancer – Patients –
        Rehabilitation.
    I. Kfir, Nira. II. Title.
    [DNLM: 1. Adaptation, Psychological. 2. Neoplasms – psychology.
QZ 200 S632c]
RC262.S55  1991
616.99′4′0019–dc20
DLC
for Library of Congress                                      91–458
                                                                CIP
ISBN 0-415-06343-4
      0-415-06344-2 (pbk)

To Vicky Clement Jones who knew instinctively how to create order out of chaos and who, after she found she had cancer, devoted her time to helping many others regain control over their lives

# Contents

Acknowledgements        ix
Foreword        xi
*Anthony Clare*
Introduction        1

1  **From victims to heroes by force of circumstance**    11

2  **The weekend seminar**    35

3  **Vicky**    97

References    136

# Contents

# Acknowledgements

We are extremely grateful to Hedy Wax and Hilary Plant, who took part in the seminars from the start. Hedy carried out all the administration and organisation of the seminars and made sure it all worked smoothly. Hilary, a specialist oncology nurse, who knew many of the patients on the ward, provided support for the patients, especially those who were ill. They gave up their weekends willingly and both continued to support people after the seminars were over, remaining friends to this day with several of the participants. Without their help these weekend seminars would not have been possible. Anne Dennison, a patient who took part in several weekend seminars together with her husband Paul, provided many ideas and valuable criticisms which went a long way to making them more responsive to the needs of the participants.

Several friends and colleagues read the manuscript and gave very helpful criticisms. We are particularly thankful to Aamer Hussein, who made important comments on the initial draft, and to Patsy Ryan and Rosie Cleghorn for their very helpful comments and criticisms. Pat Jacobson typed repeated drafts with her usual endless patience and sense of humour.

Finally, we would like to thank the patients and their relatives, who had the courage to come to the weekend seminars and have a go at challenging cancer.

# Foreword

## Anthony Clare

This is not a book about miracles nor superhuman beings coping with the unspeakable. It is about determination and commitment, rationality and common sense. In essence, it presents a dialogue between a psychotherapist and a cancer specialist illustrated by real-life accounts of individuals battling to regain a sense of control and purpose, once shattered by a diagnosis of cancer.

Over the last decade our views about cancer have changed dramatically. Once seen as the dreaded "Big C", it is now increasingly regarded as a formidable challenge – a challenge to our notions of health and disease, to our concepts of personal control, to our views of the relationship between mind and matter. In *Challenging Cancer* Nira Kfir and Maurice Slevin brilliantly describe the ways in which we can all be transformed from victims into heroes, depending on how we respond to a crisis.

It is one of the dramatic ironies of the late-twentieth century that many people are free only when they or those close to them receive a diagnosis of a disease such as cancer. And it is one of life's painful lessons that events which weaken some people strengthen others. To quote Nira Kfir, "Heroism is the most natural thing for people once they are free."

# Introduction

*Nira:* It is rare to start a book by telling the reader what the book is *not* about. But since this book is for people who know about cancer, either personally or professionally, we will try to address the first question on your mind. Can this book help cure cancer, or not? I, for one, do not know how to cure cancer and Maurice Slevin, who treats many cancer patients, does not possess any magic cure not already known and used widely. So this book is not about a cure.

The reader may switch to another alternative; is this a book about death and dying? It is not. My mother died of cancer recently and she was the only one who taught me how to die and I am not even sure when my life ends I will remember that lesson. What meaning, then, can a book of this sort have? Well, another possibility is that this is a book about miracles. This book, however, is not about miracles.

Personally, I have always hoped to experience a real miracle or at least to be enlightened. I have always known that miracles can only happen after you have lived through despair and utter hopelessness. So I hoped for a "delivery without pain" or at least a miracle to satisfy my curiosity. After practising psychotherapy for 25 years I slowly realised miracles and enlightenment do happen, and they even happen to me, only there is nothing particularly mysterious about them. They are part of a process, they stem from reason, determination and concentration. That is why this book is not about miracles, but *is* about reason, determination and concentration.

Cancer represents chaos. Chaos is the lack of central control, the lack of direction, goal and organisation. Chaos is madness within a system. Yet, new order grows out of chaos as a natural process. Having cancer creates chaos in the body, the mind and the family. Intervention – medical, psychological, social or spiritual – is aimed at trying to regain control and a sense of direction. Direction and control create movement;

movement brings hope. This book does not offer a panacea, but tries through shared experience to encourage change and movement to emerge from chaos.

This book will touch those people who, like Vicky Clement Jones, described later in this book, have "a desperate need to live".

## DISCOVERING THE CHALLENGE OF CANCER

Growing up with a mother who was very often sick and in severe pain forced me to change from a child who observes to a child always on the alert. I have never really understood what was wrong with her, but it was always more than her gall bladder attacks, migraines and other health problems with which she had learnt to live. When the attacks were over, she immediately returned to being mother, volunteer, leader, learner, reader, idealist and social activist, as if the attacks never existed.

I remember vividly one period when we moved to Holon, a new town near Tel Aviv, right after the War of Independence in 1949. Holon had more sand than a beach and less light than a village in war time. My mother's attacks always chose to come at night. There were few telephones at that time in private homes, so you had to run to fetch the doctor. Our house was far from the town centre and you had to cross an endless mountain of sand to get anywhere. Because of these difficulties, my mother never agreed to let us fetch the doctor at night. We had a ritual. Mother was in bed, the pain growing from simple aches to "deep pain" (my term for pain that was all over) and then to a situation where we could not tell if she could hear us at all. But, no matter how bad the pain, she never failed to be in control, forbidding us to call the doctor. My father and I had this ritual of: "Shall we run for the doctor, or wait for the pills to work? But what if this time they don't work and it is too late?"

So almost always, when half the night was over and my mother was much weaker, we made the decision. I ran for the doctor. Crossing the mountainous sand, barefoot in total darkness, I was paralysed by fear. I could only carry on as long as I persuaded myself my mother's life was at stake and the faster I ran the better her chances. But the worst part was yet to come. Standing sticky with sand and soaked in sweat, in front of the doctor's door, afraid to wake him and knowing that again a struggle lay ahead. The doctor, after time that felt eternal, opened the door in his pyjamas, a bit angry. "You again" was not said but felt. We argued. He suggested mother took the pills and came to see him in the morning at the clinic. I insisted it was utterly critical he came, but could never find the right words to express the urgency. I could not tell him what I knew from observation, but could not understand myself – the transformation my mother underwent after his visits. It was not just the shots he used to give her, but his presence. It did not have any impact on me since I always remembered him arguing in his half-opened pyjamas; it had a magical effect on my mother. I was mesmerised, when I finally came home with him, by the change in my mother. "Deep pain" first became local again; she was able to discuss it with him. Her beautiful face relaxed, she managed to smile. The pain that was killing her went away in front of my eyes, disappearing into the air. I always felt a miracle had been performed without anyone doing much, least of all this man with the half-open pyjamas.

It was happening in my mother's head, but it could not happen unless he came. I didn't fail, even once, to be magnetised by the process. The pills and shots did not fool me, I felt it was something more. I didn't understand it, but no-one could give me a logical explanation of what I had just experienced, the transformation from suffering to peace that happened in my mother's mind. This experience registered very deeply in my own mind, to be understood much later.

When it was all over, the last scene was played. My mother turned her head towards me and asked in a healthy, commanding voice, "Did you wash the sand off your feet?" After that sleep came blissfully.

Observing this phenomenon may partly be responsible for my choice to become a therapist. Subsequently, as a therapist, I learned change is a slow process and transformation is rare. While in medicine doctors are still waiting for the "panacea", the one remedy for all pains, psycho-therapists know one panacea cannot be found, since it must happen between us and our patients. Our panacea is an experience, or rather a series of experiences. I learnt from my childhood experiences, more than from all my later studies, that change is possible and it is up to people themselves.

When I studied for my PhD in the late 60s, in the Sorbonne in Paris, I "attended" the student revolution of May 1968. I observed, in another culture, the same phenomena of transformation. I saw my fellow students, who until May were only interested in the difference between psychoanalysis and existentialism, changing in one moment to street fighting, throwing Molotov cocktails, with messianic light in their eyes. I also saw the end of it. De Gaulle appealed to the French people on TV on a late summer afternoon, to go to the Champs-Elysées and stop the chaos. Two million people followed his voice, went out into the streets and stopped the revolution.

If it is so easy to be transformed, why is it so difficult to do it to ourselves? In all the years of study about personality, psychopathology, learning theories and even clinical practice, the therapist does not learn how to initiate change. Ideas of change yes; but how to initiate change is left to trial and error.

In 1973 when the Yom Kippur War broke out in Israel, I was asked by the Ministry of Defence, to run a rehabilitation project for bereaved families. Since I was interested in crisis situations and crisis intervention, we applied these ideas to sudden bereavements. During the years after the war, having worked with hundreds of bereaved patients, volunteers and professionals, my ideas on crisis intervention became a model that could be applied to any crisis situation.

Running workshops in crisis intervention in the United States, Greece and Great Britain, brought home the experience of the universality of all crises and the urgent need to encourage people to become interveners. In March 1986, through Maurice, I met three patients in London with advanced cancer. They had all been suffering severe anxiety and described the situation as crisis. Meeting and working with them, even though this was a single intervention, started a new course in my life. Together with Maurice, and encouraged by friends and colleagues and mostly by cancer patients and their families, we started weekend seminars in Oxford.

*Maurice:* When I was a medical student I received an excellent clinical training in all aspects of medicine. In the fifth year, training in psychiatry formed a major component of the course. This teaching concentrated on people with major psychiatric disorders such as schizophrenia, with a little instruction on the diagnosis and medical treatment of anxiety and depression. There was virtually no training even in the Department of Psychiatry or under the other medical disciplines in how to talk to patients, how to deal with talking about bad news or how to help people going through a personal crisis. Looking back, that is an incredible omission, as every doctor, in general practice or any medical specialty, has to deal with people facing the most difficult times of their lives every day of his or her career.

While some medical schools have now incorporated teaching in these areas for their students, they still remain a minority. One could say that dealing with cancer medicine is different to other medical specialties, in that our patients have particularly difficult needs. However, every specialty, medical or surgical, deals every day with cancer patients, as well as a whole variety of incurable and difficult diseases, some of which, one could argue, are considerably worse than cancer.

When I first qualified at the University of Cape Town in South Africa, the rules about telling people about cancer were very simple. You just didn't. You would use any euphemism you could find. You would talk about ulcers, shadows, lumps, but under no circumstances use the word "cancer". In fact, when talking to colleagues at the patient's bedside, one would use terms such as "non-benign disease", or "mitotic disease", to disguise the actual diagnosis. Some of the senior doctors insisted you did not write the word "cancer" in a patient's notes, because it was possible the patient might come across the notes and discover the diagnosis.

When I came to England I found that in many hospitals exactly the same system applied. Behind this tradition was the simple fact that doctors believed, and many still do, that for patients to have to face a cancer diagnosis is terrible, and by giving them the diagnosis, you can do nothing other than be destructive. Giving the diagnosis will result in people feeling despondent, hopeless, depressed and knowing that life is not worth living. This, of course, implied the doctor knew best what was right for the patient, and assumed the patient did not have any say in what they did or did not want to know. This clearly also meant the patient did not have any say in further decisions which needed to be made about the diagnosis or treatment. In all these cases, the family, husband or wife, or often the adult children, would be told the diagnosis and prognosis in detail. The family collaborated fully with the doctors in not telling the patient. Very often, when the family were told, the first thing they would say was, "Please doctor, don't tell my husband (or wife)."

So the medical profession were representing the feeling of society in general about cancer, in keeping the secret from patients. The family themselves, would, of course, tell only very, very close friends or only family members and the diagnosis would not be discussed outside their tight circle. I remember as a medical student, an intelligent, 60-year-old gentleman with a malignant mesothelioma, a cancer of the lining of the lung. He asked everybody what the diagnosis was many times. He spoke to the nurses, doctors and medical students and we all, without difficulty, because the rules were so straightforward and simple, told him he had fibrous tissue in the lung and it unquestionably had nothing to do with cancer. Seeing this gentleman over a period of months, I often felt uneasy about continuing the lie when he so clearly wanted to know what was wrong with him, but the establishment and the norm were so strong I never seriously doubted this was the right approach.

There was a clear message in this for the medical students that even doctors went along with the idea that cancer was a terrible illness, so terrible that doctors changed their tone of voice when discussing it, even at medical meetings. This rule was not absolute. Some patients, particularly those who required an operation which clearly indicated they had cancer, for example, a mastectomy for breast cancer, and some people receiving radiotherapy, were given the diagnosis. Breast cancer almost came into a separate category, largely, I suspect, because the treatment made it impossible to avoid giving the diagnosis and because knowledge about this particular cancer was much greater than others. Also, when the surgeon told a woman she had breast cancer and she had to have mastectomy, he would almost always tell her the operation would cure her, so the news could be delivered at the same time as giving a very hopeful prognosis.

I still remember, though, as a medical student, going to the radiotherapy department, feeling it was eerie, gloomy, dismal, and being left with the feeling everything about cancer was dark, unpleasant and frightening. Thinking about the common public misconceptions about cancer, it is perhaps not surprising the general public have this view. If one questions people about cancer, one finds intelligent, well-educated people believe the myths that it is always fatal, people always die prolonged, painful deaths, it may be infectious and you may pass it on to your children.

In 1978 I came to England and I started working as a registrar in the Department of Cancer Medicine at St Bartholomew's and Hackney (Homerton) Hospitals. I can clearly remember the first ward round with the consultant. We came to a patient, a man in his 40s with cancer of the colon, which had spread to the liver and lungs. We came to the bedside and the patient, who had come in the day before, looked up at the consultant and said, "Doctor, will you please tell me what is wrong with me?" The consultant sat down and told him he had cancer of the bowel, some of the cells had gone into the bloodstream and into the liver, there were some lumps in the liver and also some lumps in the lungs. He also explained he would be given drug treatment to try and shrink it. I stood at the end of the bed listening to this conversation in complete disbelief. How could this man be so cold, heartless and cruel? At the end of the ward round I went back to the patient to try to "pick up the pieces". To my utter amazement the man looked up, smiled and said, "I feel absolutely wonderful, doctor. Somebody has finally told me the truth."

He told me he had known all along he had cancer, or had at least strongly suspected it, as it was clear by the evasive way people had been treating him that there was something seriously wrong. He said that even though he was aware the outlook was poor, he somehow, paradoxically, felt relieved, happier and less frightened now he finally knew the diagnosis. This was a very interesting lesson for me. Over the years I have realised the majority of patients with cancer want to know the diagnosis and to be involved in what is happening to them. The point this gentleman made about knowing or strongly suspecting the diagnosis is one I have come across many times since. It is impossible to tell a husband or wife their spouse has cancer without expecting their behaviour to change towards that person. It is also completely unrealistic for people who have been living together for many years not to pick up subtle changes in behaviour.

One of the major giveaways is that people stop arguing. Things which previously always caused a family fight are now completely ignored. I clearly remember a man who told us he had found out his diagnosis because of the bread bin. He had been operated on for cancer of the stomach and had been told he had an ulcer. At home, while recuperating, something happened which made him realise this was not true. For the past 25 years of his marriage there had been a constant source of irritation between him and his wife. He always forgot to put the bread back in the bread bin and his wife always became irritated. After coming home from the operation he took the bread out, forgot to put it back and his wife quietly put it back without making any comment. He said when that happened he immediately knew hc had cancer.

When doctors tell the husband or wife of someone who has cancer not to tell them, and to carry on behaving normally, they are expecting the impossible. With this knowledge, one simply cannot carry on behaving in the same way, however hard one tries, and anyway this behaviour isolates the patient from those closest to him or her, at a time when their support is most needed.

Training in cancer medicine made me acutely aware of how ill at ease and uncertain I felt in dealing with many patients' questions. After some experience, talking about the diagnosis of cancer becomes relatively easy, but questions of prognosis and outlook, especially in those situations where there is no standard treatment available, frequently made me feel uncomfortable and inadequate. There were times when I would see patients and their families clearly struggling to come to terms with the information I had given them, and I felt acutely frustrated about my inability to know how best to deal with the situation. I had always thought it would be worthwhile attending courses in counselling and communication to try to help overcome this problem, but it somehow never moved to the top of my list of priorities. In 1985, however, my then wife, who was interested in relationships between parents and children, suggested we did a counselling course together. At other times I might not have taken up the suggestion and complained I was too busy, but I decided, on this occasion, to go along with the idea and we enrolled in a course for health professionals based on an Adlerian model of psychotherapy. Through this course I attended seminars by Doctor Nira Kfir, including one in Israel on crisis intervention. I found these courses stimulating, exciting and of direct relevance to my work. The event which made the greatest impression on me, however, was when I attended a further course in London on crisis intervention taken by Nira. I was asked if I could provide any "clients in crisis" for teaching purposes with the aim of helping out the organisers of the course. In the belief the patients would at least find it interesting, if not helpful, I approached three patients; two brought a spouse along and they talked to Nira, in front of a group of psychotherapists who were attending her course, about their difficulties in handling their situations.

This was the first time I had seen the use of crisis intervention applied to cancer patients directly by Nira. I was not surprised the patients found they benefited enormously from this experience. I had seen Nira work with previous patients and this was no revelation. What did come as a great surprise was the extent to which these people felt they had been helped and how, many months later, they continued to talk about how much impact this single interview had on their lives. I think Nira herself was surprised at the extent of their response. These interviews have subsequently been published as a *Crisis Intervention Verbatim* (Kfir 1988) and they, together with later experience, have demonstrated to me how ripe cancer patients and their relatives are for this sort of intervention, even when they do not see themselves as being in a crisis. Nira and I spoke at length about this experience and decided we could not ignore the observation and should try to explore it further. The result of these discussions was the concept of a weekend seminar. A dozen patients, together with a spouse or friend, met with Nira and myself at an hotel in Oxfordshire from Friday evening until Sunday afternoon, to explore the use of information, emotional support and the provision of options to help trigger change in people's lives, particularly the change in perspective from which they viewed themselves and their illness.

In the first part of this book we discuss the concept of crisis and intervention with the aims of helping cancer patients and their families, and doctors and nurses looking after cancer patients, to overcome their feelings of frustration. In the second part of the book we have tried to convey the essence and spirit of the weekend by providing an edited verbatim of a weekend seminar. The final part of the book describes the way a remarkable woman, herself a doctor, dealt with her disease when she discovered she had advanced cancer at the age of 32.

# Chapter 1

# From victims to heroes
# by force of circumstance

*Nira:* I have always felt a slight repulsion when people were referred to as victims – victims of the holocaust, rape victims, earthquake victims, Chernobyl victims, cancer victims. The concept is meant to create sympathy, but for me it carries an undertone of pity for people in a totally helpless situation. If you are not totally helpless, you are not a victim.

Whenever victims are mentioned there is always a "but". My childhood, although taking place in Jerusalem, was full of the holocaust "but" there was also the Warsaw ghetto uprising, the Partisans, the resistance, there were the children of Stalingrad. These people stood up in front of fire and cheered their comrades to turn the tide and strike back. People since the beginning of time have been fascinated by those who look death straight in the eye and fight back. Most of the time people seemed to turn a totally helpless situation to a victory by performing the most paradoxical phenomenon in life, sacrifice. While it is believed survival is the utmost motive in life, history proves otherwise. It is obvious that turning the tide from victim to hero has always been characterised by two conditions – the disappearance of fear and transferring the instinct for your own survival to an instinct for the survival of "others" – better known as altruism. It seems that life, when threatened to the utmost, creates for many a desperate need for meaning. In that instant, the meaning of life is needed more than life itself.

I believe, although heroism seems to be voluntary and out of choice, in reality it is not. Life is not lived in slow motion, where we have the time to consider and debate. A young man of 18 who threw himself on a grenade to save his comrades did not have time to debate the pros and cons of the sacrifice of his life. He was compelled to do it. He was less able than others to tolerate utter helplessness and transferred the survival instinct to the survival of others.

Why are we discussing heroism? Only because cancer victims are no different from any other victims. This book does not describe cancer patients as partisans, but there is a common denominator. When life confronts you with becoming a victim of any sort the only option left other than living your "victimhood" is becoming a hero. A hero by force of circumstance. The turn of the tide is possible, helplessness can become action, victims can become heroes. As in battle there is no way back and nothing is reversible. People become victims because of past events but become heroes when they move forward against the odds. It is possible in life, it is possible in cancer. Some do it, many more can. You cannot become a hero unless you have first become a victim. One may say only victims have hero potential.

## THE CANCER CRISIS

In the years after the Yom Kippur War in 1973, I analysed the work I had done with bereaved families and the approach I had taken. It was then I realised the crisis of bereavement is not very different from any other crisis people experience and therapists so often treat: divorce, loss, collapse of a business, war or life-threatening disease. All these events are stressful, but stress is not the same as crisis and tragedy in itself does not result in crisis. It is the interpretation one makes of the event that transforms it into a crisis. A sudden loss of a son in war is stressful and a tragedy; nevertheless, some people will mourn and suffer without experiencing crisis, while others will go into crisis.

We know crisis does not occur because of stress, since crisis does not mean using more effort, but the opposite. Faced with a stressful event to which we cannot find a solution, our energy decreases. This is different to stress and, in fact, stressful times are often looked back on with nostalgia. The reason for romantising these times is that stress, even in life-threatening situations like war, forces out the best in us. We learn to live on less sleep, less food, harder work, sharing, being alert, stretching ourselves to the limit and yet having hopes and dreams about life afterwards. In later years it is not stress for which we are nostalgic, but the high potential we discovered in ourselves at those times.

What is it that spares one person and not another from crisis? What makes the same situation a challenge for one and a dead end for another? Can it be predicted and, more importantly, can it be prevented? It was very unusual, in all my years as a therapist, that I could predict either one or the other. The "weak people" often rise to the situation and react to tragedy in a way that surprises everyone. Very often the "strong and resistant people" surprise us by breaking. This brings to mind an army experience when I was serving at a remote base in the Negev Desert. As the result of a car accident many wounded men were brought into the field hospital at the base. Volunteers with type O blood were requested. Unfortunately for me I was type O and felt compelled out of guilt to volunteer. The blood was taken in a large tent, two donors at a time. When my turn came to go in I realised that in the other bed a well-known commander of the paratroopers, who was visiting our base, was donating blood. I was eighteen-and-a-half, donating blood for the first time, and scared stiff. Needless to say his presence served only to increase my terror. My biggest fear was embarrassing myself, since I was training at that base to become an officer and fear of that sort did not seem appropriate. We both lay down, the needles were inserted and the bottles hung up over us. I calmed my hysteria, keeping half an eye all the time on the major on the next bed, hoping he would not notice my fear. But my concern was unnecessary since, exactly one minute after the needle was inserted, the major completely passed out. I cannot remember another time in my life when I felt so proud of myself as when my blood filled up that bottle. I come back to this memory every time people make predictions about "who shall survive".

The difference between challenge and crisis, victim and hero, lies in the person's understanding and interpretation of the event. If the occurrence is regarded as catastrophic, terminal and meaningless, it is unlikely we will find the courage within ourselves to struggle.

An old Persian proverb says, "To the blind, everything comes as a surprise." One of the major features of a crisis is surprise. Separation, the collapse of a business, family problems and health problems which come from neglect, are a surprise only if one is blind to the developments which led to them. Others, however, such as sudden death and serious illness diagnosed because of minor symptoms and accidents, come as a real blow. Not only do these blows stop the usual current of life, but they need immediate action, because they are critical, and create a feeling of urgency, even when the event itself is irreversible, such as death.

The suddenness, and the novelty of the situation, find us unprepared. We are used to taking advantage of our stores of knowledge and experience and shifting our minds to "automatic pilot". The automatic pilot recognises the new situation as similar to one that has occurred before and offers a ready solution. Not all life's problems, however, are dealt with by our ready solutions. We can be creative and change, finding new ways to deal with problems. Many people, indeed, don't go into crisis because they remain creative and look for new approaches when faced by unexpected, dramatic events in their lives. Whether one finds a solution depends not on the event itself, but on the interpretation one gives it.

Life always has goals beyond living itself. Only in drastic situations, critical by nature, such as concentration camps in World War II, hunger in Sudan or serious illness, does living become a goal in itself. When a sudden blow hits us and we find ourselves without ready answers and without the ability to create a response, we find our lifelong goals have dramatically lost all meaning. The old goals, such as family, welfare, success, fun, love, ambition, social involvement, changing the world, relaxation, art, power and money, have suddenly lost their charms. Faced with a situation we interpret as critical and possibly terminal, they lose meaning. This is because none of them relates to our new situation in a way that can offer solution, or often even comfort or consolation. It is almost impossible for people to live without goals and without meaning. Even surviving, just for survival's sake, must have a meaning to make us strive for it. Dramatic events, or personal catastrophes, even if they happen in one area of life, such as health, love, finance, if interpreted as a catastrophe, rather than as a problem, cause people to lose meaning and trust, not only in this area of life, but in the whole of life. One may say people generalise the hopelessness they feel in one area or towards one relationship, to the totality of life. When that happens, there is a sense of emptiness and powerlessness. A 16-year-old girl kills herself after the boy she loves left her and asked another girl to the village dance. She "knows" she can never love any man again, and, what is more, no man will ever love her. This is critical and terminal to her and life has lost all meaning. The realisation is "reality" to her. The lack of a goal is a lack of hope and unless one can find that hope again, life appears useless.

It is believed the winning of any battle depends heavily on "fighting spirit". The two concepts, fight and spirit, seem to belong to two totally different areas of life. Our image of "fight" is one of movement, our legs running or kicking, our hands hitting or using tools and our head using all our senses to guide the movement. The posture of fight is one of power. "Spirit" is associated with calmness, no movement, a relaxed body, eyes closed as in prayer or meditation. The power here is of a different sort, an unseen power. But the combination of the two creates a new image which is neither fight nor spirit; it means self-recharging, determination and hope.

The young girl just described is a person at the point of defeat. At this point she experiences herself as totally powerless. Defeat is not just losing, it is rather the way a person feeds back to themselves the defeat, as eternal, terminal and hopeless.

Crisis is, then, a realisation that there is no hope, no power, and the situation is critical and possibly terminal. It is the realisation that one is lost, unprepared, out of orbit, with no guidance. It is sudden and dangerous. Life's goals are lost. There is an inability to visualise the future, other goals or new meaning. When all these occur, a person is in crisis.

## CHARACTERISTICS OF THE CANCER CRISIS

Most people, though, experience crisis rarely, and many people, never. Nevertheless, the symptoms of crisis may appear in any critical situation, such as discovering you have cancer, or being a spouse of a cancer patient. Many people who participated in our weekend seminars claimed they cannot remember being in crisis when their cancer was diagnosed or recurred and neither did they remember their friends or fellow patients experiencing a crisis. If we want to relate to cancer as a crisis and to suggest a crisis intervention approach, it is essential to establish our belief that the diagnosis of cancer starts a process that has all the characteristics of crisis. Cancer is almost always a sudden realisation that finds us unprepared. Even cancer specialists, who are most knowledgeable about cancer, do not feel prepared when they, themselves, develop cancer. The suddenness is surprising, even after a long process of examination, anxiety and suspicion. The diagnosis usually finds one without previous experience of this situation, and without personal solutions. This is also true when a recurrence is diagnosed. After one has learnt to cope with having cancer, having treatment and establishing hope, recurrence is a totally new situation bearing little resemblance to the initial diagnosis. The major issue, when cancer occurs, is the realisation that the hope you built up, and the faith you had in your previous treatment, prove false. You now search, afraid, for a new attitude and a new sort of hope.

Cancer, at first, makes people "look again" at their priorities in life. For many, it is not just another look, but creates a strong need to change priorities. It is like being given an opportunity to look at life from a higher level, a photograph taken by a satellite. The pattern, the plan, is much clearer than before. This new view of life makes the old goals seem doubtful, if not meaningless.

The concept of crisis, as applied here to cancer, results from the catastrophic interpretation of a tragedy as a TRAGEDY. The web of crisis that envelops a person is spun by the lack of information, the lack of a sense of support, and the lack of new options.

## LACK OF INFORMATION

What do we mean by "a lack of information"? There is nothing more paradoxical than the "sudden" realisation there has been a cancer growing in your body. You realise the cancer has been a slow secretive development. One person put it this way, "I felt while I was living my life, the cancer was living its own. It had made room for itself and grown at the expense of other parts of my body", or, as somebody else said, "It felt like Rome, unaware and oblivious of the Huns about to invade."

This discovery, that there has been a process going on in our bodies, unknown to us, creates the first confusion and sometimes shock. People's reactions vary from "Cancer! But I have always lived a clean life", to "But I am 100 per cent fit." This new, startling information starts a whole process of awareness of the lack of information we have about ourselves. Before you have had time to assimilate this lack of awareness about your disease and your body, you face another un-known: the treatment for cancer. Cancer therapies such as surgery, radiotherapy and chemotherapy, although well known by name, are mysterious and confusing, and the outcome is equally uncertain. The problem is, this information is not totally new. A complete lack of information is often easier to deal with than partial information or misinformation. While the suggestion of treatment gives you hope, you also "know" from your "previous life" before becoming a cancer patient that cancer is "death", and treatment is painful, slow, ugly and helpless. While previously you felt fully in control of your life, you now realise there is a lot you don't know or understand. At the same time you have to make critical decisions, life and death decisions. About twenty or thirty years ago, before the information age we now live in, it may, in a way, have been easier for patients. There was little doubt you could trust honourable and learned experts, such as doctors. In even older times, before science replaced religion, you trusted God to protect you. Para-phrasing John Naisbitt in *Mega-trends*, (Naisbitt 1988) we first had the industrial revolution, then the scientific revolution and we now live in the information revolution, where information is the most vital and sought-after item.

Information is vital because it means control and power. Throughout the life of someone with cancer new questions will arise all the time and new information will be needed. The problems divide mainly into two categories: those which require practical information in order for concrete decisions to be made, and those that concern our feelings about life and its meaning. Practical problems do not always have simple black and white solutions and problems with the meaning of life often cannot be solved by tackling the issues directly. Information is not always simple; it may be conflicting and confusing. Double messages abound. "I should trust my doctor and his suggestions – I should go for a second opinion." We know how important it is to trust and fully co-operate with your doctor, and how important it may be not to delay treatment; but on the other hand we hear people talking about incorrect diagnoses, which may cost us our lives. Most of these stories will be fiction and rumour, but some are real, so we worry about whether a second opinion should be obtained. It is not just the "expertise" of the doctor that is important, but his or her personality and manner. Doctors with a good reputation may not be skilled in human relationships. The person with whom you are entrusting the most important decisions in your life may not include the whole of "you" in the process. He or she may relate only to the "cancerous you". "My doctor does not relate to me as a person who has cancer, but as a cancer that has a person." The doctor may be uncommunicative and provide little information. Are you going to educate your doctor, or do you have to look for another one? How easy is it to find a doctor who understands:

> I need my doctor to explain to me, to be cheerful, to share his experience and guide me, not only in the treatment, but with my feelings as well. I need my doctor to discuss the possibility of death, and to find options that are unknown to me, because, without him, I don't even know where to look for them. I would also like to feel free to talk to him about trying alternative treatments, without fear of his resentment or contempt, that would destroy my hope and enthusiasm, or spoil the relationship.

This confusion, and difficulty in making decisions, add to the sense of a lack of information and a feeling of helplessness.

*Maurice:* People are often afraid to ask their doctors for a second opinion. They worry the doctor will be offended and feel his or her professional ability has been questioned. When people are very anxious it is often useful to suggest directly that they have a second opinion, rather than wait for them to ask. A second opinion gives a person the opportunity to talk to someone else who will present the information in his or her own way and, by hearing things from a different point of view, it may help to clarify and reassure. It is uncommon for major differences of opinion to exist among cancer specialists about the main policy of management. Most differences of opinion that may exist are not crucial to the final result or chance of cure and they exist in areas where the answers are not known. If this is explained to people, they are usually able to accept it. Problems occur with second opinions when you get conflicting information. The patient then has to make a decision and often has not enough experience on which to base this decision. He or she then needs a third opinion and so on. On the other hand, some people have a need to see many doctors in the beginning of their search for information and second opinions are just part of that process. Many people do not have enough background knowledge to understand the medical journals and second opinions are a simple, practical way of obtaining further information. The only times I have seen second opinions make a real difference is when patients have been told by doctors, who are not specialists in cancer, that they are incurable when, in fact, this is incorrect. Every cancer doctor can quote patients of this sort, even though they are uncommon.

I will relate two stories which are good examples of this rare situation. A 55-year-old lady with inoperable ovarian cancer was told by a general surgeon there was no available treatment and she should be treated with medicines to control her symptoms only. Her husband was devastated and had no reason to disbelieve the opinion, but felt that, for his own peace of mind, he wanted a second opinion with an oncologist. She was referred to me. We treated her with the standard treatment for ovarian cancer and she had a complete remission with eradication of all the disease. Six years have passed since she finished her treatment and she is almost certainly cured.

Seven years ago I saw a 27-year-old woman with a malignant thymoma, a very rare type of cancer, who had been told by a surgeon she had 3 months to live and no treatment was available. This opinion was simply incorrect. We treated her with the intensive, standard therapy of chemotherapy and radiotherapy. She had a complete remission and remains well, free of disease and, once again, is almost certainly cured. She has just married and writes to me regularly. These are rare examples, but I believe everyone should have the opportunity of seeing a cancer specialist before accepting the opinion that no treatment is available for their cancer.

*Nira:* Many other questions arise, whether or not to tell your friends and, maybe more critically, your boss. How much do you tell your family, especially young children or elderly parents? There is much to be said for unloading your burden by talking to people, but you know that telling people will create a change in their attitude towards you. You are tempted to let things stay the way they were before you knew you had cancer. As long as you don't tell, you can live a part-time fantasy relating to people as if cancer does not exist. Again, there is no right or wrong attitude, the question is only, what is the cost to you? If you find you are getting away from people, hiding, then you should at least be aware that distance from friends may sometimes be irreversible. Often you may feel it is not a priority for you, right now, to educate your friends about cancer and change their attitudes. But if you fail to do this, their anxieties may cause them to move away. So by force of circumstance a cancer patient finds him- or herself educating friends. If your son joins the Hari Krishna, you may initially be in a state of shock, having heard only negative things about the organisation. However, should he continue, you may find yourself, somewhat reluctantly, educating yourself and explaining to others the bright side of it.

Information is, by definition, neither "good" nor "bad". It is open to different interpretations by different people, at different times. Being given a diagnosis of cancer will have a different impact on someone who is 20 years old than on someone who is 60 years old. The information people need is different when they are first diagnosed to that required when the cancer recurs or is cured. Our experience has been that, after an initial period following diagnosis, people need information about symptoms, treatment, side effects, Social Security and means of adapting to the changes in their life. Those who have had a recurrence may be disillusioned by their initial enthusiasm and hope and the advice they first received. Although they stay with their doctor, they may become more interested in experimental treatments, or natural remedies, faith healing or spiritual guidance.

People cured of cancer may still have a need to understand it all or tell the world about it. Not everyone follows particular tracks, but for every individual, different information is needed at different stages. Why does information have so much impact? Critical events throw our life into chaos. Becoming unemployed after 30 years is not just a matter of not having a job; it is a total change in the way you spend your days, your self-esteem, your respect for the system and your family. In brief, the whole of your life is unfamiliar and chaotic. Having more information about being unemployed may have a strong therapeutic influence that may move you to action, rather than hiding at home. Information is a major asset when trying to create a new order and less chaos. Although it is a common belief that information and knowledge are a "post mortem" on life ("What good can this information do me if it cannot change the facts?"), information can change how you relate to the facts; it changes how you act and the way you behave. The effect information has on people depends on their situation and varies widely. There is information that helps you understand, gives you insight and stimulates you to act. Other information relaxes you and helps things fall into place. If information can be so valuable, why is it so many people have to be encouraged to look for it and don't do it intuitively? Is it just laziness or the inertia that overtakes us as we get older? Not necessarily. Observing people's rejection of information shows this has its private logic as well.

## INFORMATION ANXIETY

A Japanese anti-nuclear activist described at an international conference on reactions to stress what he called the "Hiroshima effect". If you show people a film about Hiroshima with close-ups of the victims, the more horrible the pictures, the less effective they are. The horror and helplessness cannot be tolerated. The message is rejected, together with the horror that created it. In trying to reach large numbers of people, one must find a practical way of giving a little of the horror to create a sense of "I can do something about it" rather than a sense of helplessness. Rejecting information is denial. What is really being denied is the sense of helplessness. That is why, although we suggest cancer patients should search for information, it is important you have the ability to translate information into possibilities, rather than despair. We can never handle all the information relevant to any particular point in our life. That is why denial is basically healthy. We must not try to contrast denial with information, since they are not contradictory. Denial is a break we need to assimilate new facts.

My last check-up showed a slight rise in my blood cholesterol. While gathering information about this "new part of me", cholesterol, I called a friend of mine, a very knowledgable doctor. Her reaction was something like this: "Oh! This is not very good, you know what it means, it increases your chances of having a heart attack, blockage in another artery, like having a stroke, a blockage of ...." I felt if I didn't stop this conversation, I might soon hear I was more likely to get syphilis or Alzheimer's or ...! I tried to defend myself, saying I had already started to take fish oil. She laughed and said, "Of course, but do you know how many tablets you need daily to make it effective?" Afterwards I felt very low. This information may be correct, only it does not encourage; it has the "Hiroshima effect". Luckily, I balanced this conversation by talking to another friend, not an expert on cholesterol, who said:

A raised cholesterol is not necessarily to do with your diet, since you have been a vegetarian for many years, and generally avoid fat. These levels are not very worrying, a few years ago they were regarded as being within the normal limit. This is not something to worry seriously about, but if you make changes in your diet, take some medication and exercise, in a month or two, your cholesterol level will drop. This is very common, it may even do you a lot of good.

I almost became cheerful about this new opportunity, listening to him.

People whose task it is to give information to people under stress, like doctors, therapists, family or friends, are not always naturally gifted to do the job. No wonder many patients have the "don't tell me" reaction, followed by, "Just tell me what I should do." Although millions of pounds are spent providing clear, encouraging printed and broadcast information, there is a great need for personalised information given by someone who cares for you and stimulates your desire to learn. This is not common. Books, films, stories of other people, provided we can identify with them personally, can provide information to change our mood from passive acceptance or denial to search and action.

Danielle, a 32-year-old woman, came to live in Israel as a Kibbutz volunteer when she was 25. She met Yossi, a Kibbutz member, and two years later they were married. Danielle became the English teacher for grammar school children. She used different methods to make the children curious about and interested in the English language. She, herself, was a learner, a person who was always looking for new ways. She completely changed the approach to the learning of language in this Kibbutz school. When she was 30, she became pregnant with Nataly. Every now and then she came close to fainting. After the birth she became very depressed. It was only her husband's trust in her natural zest for life that made the doctor look further than the depression. Soon a rare brain tumour was discovered. Danielle's attitude, right from the beginning, was characterised by the need to know and find out. She went on being the learner she had always been. Three months after her operation, when she was struggling with recovery, hormones and taking care of her baby, her husband came to see me. The reason was information. Danielle had ordered a book about rare brain tumours and he went to collect it. On the bus coming home, he opened the book and the first thing he saw was a table describing the prognosis for each cancer. Yossi searched for "their" cancer and there, right in front of his eyes, it said "maximum survival – 14 months". This was his first confrontation with the reality of this tumour. He was shocked. He did not give the book to Danielle, but came to see me.

Danielle died 14 months after her operation. In this brief time, she underwent two small operations and treatments including experimental therapy. She also went abroad for another opinion. She followed a diet, tried as much as possible to swim and read, or made others read to her, all the information she could find. She came to see me whenever her condition allowed to discuss the question of Nataly's future. Danielle read that book, studied the prognostic table and wanted to prove it wrong.

She comes to mind more than any other person, when I think about the need for information. I tell the story particularly because the obvious question is, "What good did it do her to know?" To her, knowing was vital, because control over her condition was absolutely essential. Control may not overcome cancer, but helps us, while we live, to be alive. Crisis should be looked on NOT as a tragedy, but as an opportunity.

We used the term "heroism" at the beginning of this chapter. History is full of heroes, remembered not because of the outcome of the heroic conduct. Some won, many didn't, but even though they didn't win, they and their people stopped being victims and had the freedom to act. Danielle did exactly the same. During most of those 14 months, Danielle heroically learnt, adapted, tried to be optimistic and arranged for the future. And yet, like all "great events", when you are close enough, it doesn't seem anything but natural. We suggest in this book that heroism, created by force of circumstance, is a natural act for people who find themselves victims.

One may say that, after her operation, Danielle became preoccupied with the present and the future. She was not in crisis, even when the situation was, indeed, critical. She refused to be helpless, she adapted to a new behaviour rather than switching to "automatic pilot", and did not feel defeated, almost to the end of her life. When there were no more present goals, she switched to goals in the future, tried to get meaning from the fact that her wishes for the future, for Nataly, would be respected.

Many people are greatly helped by seeking for information all the time, an on-going act of search. Knowledge, not just for its own sake, but because it suggests new options to us is likely to require more information. New information leads to new options, and using these options makes the change. Helpful information is associated with solutions, options and control. The rest will be forgotten anyway.

Yael was 42 years old. Since her teens she was said to be anxious and a hypochondriac. She became a teacher, quite successful at her work and social life. The great part of her time, however, was spent seeing doctors, since her anxiety grew with time and, in spite of her general fitness, she always felt there was something very wrong with her. When Yael met Shlomi, she started to feel anxious about having a baby. She married Shlomi and very soon found out she, indeed, could not have a baby. Since the waiting list for adoption was very long and when their time came they would be too old, they opted for a South American adoption. They invested all their money and planned to leave for Brazil. Waiting to go, Yael went for a general check-up out of habit or boredom. A lump was found in her breast. She was so anxious that she required medication. After a mastectomy she started chemotherapy and responded well.

For the first time in her life she was almost free of anxiety. The relief was so powerful, it overshadowed the difficulty of the treatment. Yael was able, for the first time in her life, to discuss her future with her doctors openly. To her husband's amazement, the doctor told her she had a 50–50 chance of survival and she accepted it and felt hopeful. At the end of her treatment she told me she had made up her mind definitely to go to Brazil and adopt a child.

In the beginning her doctor thought she was challenging his trust in her likelihood of recovery by discussing it with him. But she was no longer an anxious person, obsessed with a catastrophic view of life, searching for a guarantee for eternal life or health. Now, Yael was alive and without fear. She lived in South America and adopted a beautiful son. She and her husband have now joined parents' groups for "mid-life parents of small children", opting for every opportunity to live a better and richer life.

The story of Yael was chosen so we could look at the different aspects of what happened to her and what she did. Her decision to adopt a child at that point in her life did not win general approval. Members of her family felt unable to express their concern about the child, or the father, should she not recover. They also believed, as many other people do, that she should now devote all her energy to her own recovery, "You now have only yourself to consider." Early in this chapter, we discussed the need for goals and meaning, as being essential to life. Also, that a person's major goal in life cannot be him- or herself, except when life is threatened and survival is the only goal that matters.

Victor Frankl, psychiatrist and author of *Man's Search For Meaning* (Frankl 1959), survived the Nazi concentration camps and describes this very situation, when he tells us that those who survived the camps were the people who had a sense of meaning attached to their lives and a belief in the role they had to fulfil in this life. He claims when put to the most horrible tests, people found that striving for meaning, rather than for survival itself, was the greatest goal in human life. People are often told, at times of illness, bereavement or old age, "You must take care of yourself." At the prime of life, we often have hardly any time for ourselves and wish to have more time for "me". When this time comes, it is frequently part of loneliness, emptiness or old age. It is striving that is the essence of meaning and you cannot strive for yourself. Striving can only be for another person you love, a task you undertake, an interest you have, or, in Victor Frankl's words, "leaving your finger-prints on the world".

Cancer forces one, for a time, to be preoccupied with treatment, concern for your own welfare and anxieties. But after a period of assimilating this new knowledge, one starts to look at life from a different level, to feel a need for change. What people learn is not to take life for granted, an understanding that in itself creates a new perspective on life. Many people who have to live with cancer for the first time discover "The sky is blue, I am really only seeing it for the first time." These "revelations" are very real to them. The awareness of life becomes more acute as you become more conscious of yourself; you also become more conscious of the world and other people. That is when the search starts. The threat to your life posed by cancer sends you searching in many different directions.

People commonly resist these urges, because they are anxious they will disturb the balance in their lives. The "new", although tempting, is also frightening. It is even more alarming to the people who live with you. They fear, realistically, that the changes in you will affect their lives as well. Cancer is an enormous change in your life. It is forced on you, but once they have come to terms with it, many people feel a real need for change.

## INFORMATION AND CHANGE

When I use the term "many people", it is not just from reluctance to generalise, but rather because there is no single approach to suit everyone. There are people, living with cancer, who only want their life to return to how it was before. This wish, to wake up and find oneself one day before the nightmare started, is very characteristic of crisis. People will struggle mainly to re-establish their life as it was before they had cancer.

I have observed this with many people after the Yom Kippur War in 1973. Some could not get on with life and cherished the past, despite realising the changes that had occurred were irreversible. Others had a strong urge to make greater use of their new life. We were surprised to find the incidence of divorce in bereaved parents was much higher than expected. We were surprised because there is a common belief that tragedy brings people closer. Indeed it may, but only for those who have been close before. Those who were not find it difficult to go on together after tragedy. Crisis often brings the close closer and makes the distant more distant. The realisations that accompany and precede change are alarming to many people.

Suzy and David's 3-year-old daughter died of leukaemia. They had marital difficulties before, but after the pain of this loss, they simply needed to get away from each other, and so, one month after their daughter's death, David moved out. Jonathan, at the age of 56, was diagnosed as having advanced cancer. He had been married for 32 years to a woman he had never loved, but never before considered leaving. He shocked his family and friends when he announced his separation from his wife. He realised for the first time, faced with advanced cancer, he had never really had the freedom to control his life. Now, he wanted to use this freedom and so left.

To the impartial observer, these stories evoke a response like, "Poor guy, what a shame, he was probably shattered by the diagnosis." In reality this is not true. The "poor guy", just like Yael, found himself, for the first time in his life, without fear. The need for new options in people who have had cancer varies from searching for a cure, to changing their lifestyle, including food, exercise, sport, music, art and the need for expression. Crisis stops movement and all people want is to be protected by their family, to hide from life. Once you have moved through the crisis, the change that occurs generally draws you towards living a fuller life. There is no doubt, people who allow themselves to follow their sense of "there is more to life than I have experienced so far" find the struggle easier, have a new-found sense of control and feel more positive about themselves and life itself. It is often said that having a positive attitude enhances the likelihood of curing cancer itself. Nobody knows if this is true, but there is no doubt it enables you to get more life out of life.

New concepts enter one's life – relaxation, meditation, stress reduction, exercise, psychology, family relationships and positive thinking. There is choice between "back to normal" i.e. BC (before cancer), or "moving on", which means change. Yael experienced the rare insight that happens to people who have realised their most horrible fear has just come true. This is a moment carrying the sense of "beyond fear". All the energy people invest in fear is released to be used for life itself. That is a time when people make their "jumps" in life. Yael, who had been so preoccupied all her life with the fear of death, felt free, free of the opinions of her family and of what people thought of her. Vicky Clement Jones dared to use the expression, "Cancer freed me." Each person uses this new-found freedom in a different way. Cancer, in itself, is not freedom, it is more often closer to slavery, but freedom emerges when you discover the uselessness of fearing for your life when you may, in fact, be dying and discover the futility of many lifelong concerns that limited you. To be free to live only means using more options in your life and enlarging your choice.

What encourages people to look actively for further options is mostly other people. Whether they are family, friends, experts or just strangers, each can be the trigger you need. The *Encyclopaedia of Psychology* (Corsini 1984) defines crisis intervention as a human condition that compels other people to interfere. Different people and cultures take different views about how much interference they welcome, but this encyclopaedic description still holds and is universal.

## SUPPORT – THE DOUBLE MESSAGE

Once again, we are faced with a paradox. Just as the need for information can be critical, so is the need for support, but just as people have to be encouraged to seek information, people have to be encouraged to ask for support as well. "Do it yourself" is the great message of our individualistic society, so asking for help can be very distressing. For many people, asking for help means weakness, dependence and proof that you cannot take care of yourself. People who opt for using psychotherapy admit this decision was not taken lightly, since they always believe they can take care of themselves. It is as if using someone else's wisdom, expertise, energy, good will and love minimises your own.

The mere term, "support", repulses many people. And yet, what proves to be most valuable at times of crisis is exactly this. Another person's view, or their different experience or simply their effort to help you, can make the difference. There are three main groups of potential supporters: family and friends, experts and strangers.

## SUPPORT BY FAMILY AND FRIENDS

Family, parents, spouses, brothers and sisters, are the first line of support. Their help ranges from physical to financial to spiritual: accompanying such patients to treatments, taking care of them, doing for them what they used to do for themselves. Getting help from one's family is, most of the time, quite natural. But to many, this requires a lot of adaptation. Many people cannot tolerate intrusion into their privacy, dependence or the change in their role in the family. If you have always been the supporter, whether the problem solver or breadwinner, you may find it bizarre to become dependent on those whom you had previously expected to support. Although a family is often said to be a system of division of labour and mutual support, this is not how it functions in practice. There is no such thing as equal division of responsibility. Mainly because people are unique in the way they handle life's tasks. Not only because of the stereotypical roles of men and women, children and parents, siblings, but also because all relationships never take an equal share, either in love or duties. In difficult times this becomes accentuated. There is always one child more concerned than the others, one sibling more sensitive to the needs of others. Equality is a matter of human rights. In families or in any other group, people are unique. Each person contributes in a different way and, whatever our expectations, some people closest to us can be of little help on a rainy day. When the person who is the natural supporter of the family, often the mother, has cancer, the situation calls for a great deal of adaptation. Professor Atara Dinur, from the Hadassa Medical Centre in Jerusalem, found that the family member who suffers most is the husband of a wife who has cancer.

Family support is not only natural, but is expected by society. A neglected child will be asked, "Where are your parents?" But most people who come for therapy are struggling through family relationships whether past or present. (A great number of murders occur within families themselves.) Faced with the need to be taken care of by your family is not a rosy prospect for everyone. Also, for many today, a close family within reasonable distance is non-existent. So we must accept that, for many people, help may be needed beyond the family limits. Families, when someone has cancer, often put aside all other concerns. This asks for sacrifice. It starts right after diagnosis, since from then on it is not only the patient's life that is affected, but very often that of his or her spouse or family to an even greater extent. With the new division of roles, sometimes new discoveries are made. A relevant question would be, "Who will support the supporter?"

Laura, 28, is the wife of Sam, 32, who was diagnosed as having cancer right after they had their first baby. She said:

For months, I did nothing but take care of the baby, and Sam. Both were demanding and obsessed with their needs. The baby declared its needs aloud, while Sam declared his by being depressed and hopeless. He used all his energy for his job, and came home, only to be depressed and hide. Home became his shelter. It was never said, but understood, that joy, fun, light-heartedness, or anything indicating future plans, were in bad taste. Also any complaint of a mundane nature seemed ridiculous in comparison to Sam's cancer.

Laura developed a sense of being victimised by her husband and baby. It seemed wrong to neglect Sam because he had cancer and she resented the baby. It seemed unfair that the only person in the house who had a right to enjoy life and have a future was the baby. Laura, who was young, healthy and alive, felt trapped. She sensed, or imagined, Sam envied her need for sex, fun and diversion. He often said, "How silly people are when they spend their energy on anything less than solving world problems, such as the prevention of disease." Laura felt this was directed at her and as time passed, she even sensed Sam wished it on her.

She started to struggle for her own survival. She sneaked out for a run or a swim in the pool. To escape at night she went once a week to her tap-dancing lessons. She clung to life, secretly. In the end Sam realised how much they were drifting apart, and suggested to Laura they look together for help and counselling.

The supporter may find him- or herself, as Laura did, in the "victim" role. While people are always concerned, encouraging and helpful to the patient, the supporter needs to create his or her own support network. This may also be extended to the whole family. Richard and Susan are an example. When Richard was initially diagnosed with cancer, he could not tolerate it at all. He developed an acute anxiety which had to be treated. During this time he clung to Susan. He would not allow her to leave the house. She was his connection to life when he could not tolerate other people or any subject other than his cancer and prospects of cure. Susan was a churchgoer. Richard had never shown any interest in the church, but tolerated and respected her involvement. Now, facing cancer, Richard lost interest in all people but Susan, who practically lived his life, his cancer, his anxiety. The house was closed to the outer world. The only activity Susan kept going to was her church. For the first time she realised what a strong support it was for her. It seemed odd, for a person who had believed all her life the church was supportive, to realise it really was so. The church had two different meanings. One was religion, faith and God: the other was the people – people with whom she had shared many things over a period of years – chorusing, Sunday school, charity events, but who were never invited to each other's homes. They were "church friends only". Now, it felt natural to her to have these friends, rather than anyone else, come to the house and become Richard's friends as well. Susan clung to the church in the same way Richard clung to her. This was her hope, her meaning, her support.

Even in a close-knit family, like Laura and Sam, or Richard and Susan, support does not necessarily come from within the family, either for the supporters or even for the patient. Not many people are "trained" by life to become "cancer patients". This means many don't know how, or even want to use other people for support. There seems to be a whole variety of attitudes to the "other person" in our society. Simone de Beauvoir, lifelong friend of Jean-Paul Sartre, described in her diaries a relevant story. Sartre was touring France and giving presentations on his existential philosophy to audiences who ranged from large meetings in the city to small rural communities. He was trying to interpret his philosophy to the "person in the street". From my own experience of being "Sartre's student" in Paris in the late 1960s, I doubt very much it was possible to interpret "Sartre for the masses". Simone de Beauvoir describes a talk Sartre gave in a rural community to a small group of people. He had tried to explain his concept of "the other" versus "the authentic me". At the end of his talk, complete silence fell on the room. The situation was saved by an elderly lady, who stood up and said, "Mr Sartre, if I understood you correctly, the 'other person' is hell, if so, am I right in believing 'I' am paradise"? This lady, in her naive way, had actually caught the bull by the horns. In fact, all existential philosophers believe the need for others is "hell" and the only way to achieve happiness is to be self-sufficient and depend on oneself. Relating this to our discussion about supporters, how can we trust supporters if the "other" is hell and the world is an enemy camp?

Jews and Christians, among other religions, teach love for God and for your neighbours. Humanistic psychology, through giant thinkers like Alfred Adler, Eric Fromm, Abraham Maslow and Viktor Frankl, teaches that mutual dependence is crucial and the meaning of life lies in the "other". Contributing to others is what makes us "human". Humanistic psychology, therefore, is at the opposite extreme from Sartre and suggests "love thy neighbour", contribute, give, care and even sacrifice yourself for your people and your causes.

So the concept of support is confused in 20th-century thinking, but whenever it is discussed, it means to "give" support, rather than to receive support. It is, in fact, much easier to give support than to get it and it often requires us to retrain, to know how to receive and use support ourselves. To many people, needing support means weakness. Organisations, like countries at war, are not ashamed to ask for support. It is accepted to be "needy together", and to be needy for a cause, rather than for oneself. For many, even the first circle of help, the family, is an obstacle. People feel uneasy about disturbing, embarrassing or using their family. In reality, being asked to help is confirmation one has meaning in the person's life and evidence that your unique ability is considered useful. But even asking for help doesn't always mean you know how to use that help. What is help? To help means to create new possibilities for another person. Whether this is helping with medical or nursing care, or caring for someone's baby, or helping lift someone's depression by creating hope, or providing scholarships for the education of people who could not otherwise afford it, or hiding the Jews from the Nazis or organising a deprived community, they all have one thing in common: they create new possibilities.

People who become ill with cancer often feel their situation is one that does not have possibilities. In situations like this, people feel they have used up all their possibilities. They believe if they cannot see the possibilities, nor will anyone else. To ask for help, physically or spiritually, means only to consider new possibilities. For many, just asking for help is already a new possibility. When Maurice and I started to run weekend seminars for cancer patients and supporters, we were concerned that once we offered this facility, there would be too many people who wanted to come and we would not be able to cope with the demand. But this didn't happen. We, like many other "help organisa-tions", realised "support" does not sell well. One has to promote it, or rather inspire a new attitude in order to encourage people to learn about new attitudes. How "help" helps is still unknown. To change from being depressed and hopeless to being hopeful and energetic, sometimes through a brief encounter with an individual, is a fact, but it cannot be explained. Why is it that certain information given by one person is just "information", whereas the same information given by another is "help"? With cancer, one needs all kinds of new possibilities and no-one can find them all on their own.

## SUPPORT – PROFESSIONAL HELP

We discussed earlier the three major sources of support: family and friends, experts and others. While family and friends are the obvious source of support and are triggered naturally to help, the situation is often much more difficult when one tries to get help from the experts. Earlier, Maurice described how variable doctors' attitudes are to cancer patients' general state of wellbeing. The issues of hope, change, encouragement and exploration beyond treatment, are really a doctor/ patient relationship issue. Bernie Seigal in his book, *Love, Medicine and Miracles*, discusses the concept of the "exceptional patient". What makes a patient an "exception" is not being important, rich or influential, although these may create more impression in the beginning; the "exceptional" patient is one who triggers and stimulates in the doctor a new kind of interest and creativity, rather than the "automatic pilot" reaction to your cancer. People who treat others, such as doctors or psychotherapists, always have memories of a few patients who taught them to think in new ways, try a new approach or become more helpful themselves. These patients are often not the celebrities, but rather a "Mrs Smith" or "Mr Jones", courageous, direct, searching people, not ashamed of their own ideas. Exceptional patients don't indulge in "Should I say this to my doctor?" but become their doctor's colleague and create the therapeutic partnership.

The sense of helplessness many cancer patients feel often starts at the consultation with the doctor. It is there and then the patient needs to encourage him- or herself to be free, to speculate, to search, to ask, to challenge and to offer his or her own experience. It is often found that the "exceptional patient" brings out the "exceptional doctor" in us.

The story of Hannah is one I will never forget. Hannah lost her two sons in the Yom Kippur War. A series of suicide attempts were her reaction to this double loss. She could not accept the possibility of help from anyone, could not believe life would continue, let alone have any meaning. She was referred to me, or rather I was referred to her, since she didn't leave her home. In spite of the fact that we established an immediate rapport and I become her therapist, a friend and a family member, in reality, not much changed. By the end of the first year she still felt suicide was a better option than life. My attitude was new to me. I felt trapped between my own inability and incompetence on the one hand and the growing admiration I had for this person on the other. My admiration was not because of her death wish, but rather because of her logical thinking, her straightforwardness and, above all, her absence of fear. She was the patient, but at the same time she was also the observer. She had never before had any close relationship with the medical profession, or with psychotherapy. In a family community, she was always the person people turned to for help and support. Now, when she was in the role of the patient, she went on to be a learner, only she now studied us. She used to tell the psychiatrists, in a friendly way, about her disappointment with psychiatry. She said it never occurred to her psychiatry merely consisted of giving pills, or, as she put it, "I always thought psychiatry was related to the psyche, not to chemistry." She wondered why the psychiatrists had no more information about life than she did, how they could not help her regain the desire to live. She felt all they were doing was giving her pills, which gave a dry taste to the mouth and were not going to be helpful. Hannah did not criticise the doctors, she just observed and understood and even tried to encourage them and help. She won everyone's admiration and, at the same time, all of us, general practitioners, psychiatrists and myself, felt more and more impotent. She asked us to give her a reason to get up in the morning, not a tranquilliser. A common way out for therapists in this kind of impasse is to retreat and take cover under professional distance and diagnosis, to use other labels for the patient. If she does not respond, she becomes another one that did not respond to psychotherapy.

Only there was something in Hannah forcing me not to give up. Together we started a search for meaning in her life. Psychology did not offer much beyond understanding, so I felt compelled to look elsewhere. We went to talk to the army Chief Rabbi. This was a beginning. We looked for another doctor, who changed her medication, and we looked for a different sort of doctor as well. We found him. When she went to see him, late in the evening in a small apartment, to her utter amazement, she found him standing on his head, exercising. She was not used to people who didn't jump to attention when treating her, so this was refreshing. He suggested she practise the Feldenkreis Technique, based on exercise and posture. This was a new language and something in his manner created a feeling of hope. He referred her to a homeopath, another new language. None of these people, the rabbi, the doctor, the homeopath, felt guilty or responsible for her condition. Neither were they impotent. Each had a belief in his "one cure" for life's problems. Slowly she started to accept she was perhaps not in a "dead-end situation" and by searching, slowly regained meaning in her life. She was not able to stand on her head, although she tried. She did not become a vegetarian, although she tried. She did not become religious, although she also looked into this. But the search, the devoted rabbi, the unusual doctor, the homeopath, each a strong believer in his own solutions, created a hunger in her for her own search and offered her the opportunity to find herself and to become, as she later did, a poet.

For me, Hannah was a landmark, in being able to understand people better and not being afraid or trapped by convention. I learnt through her to look for more than I could offer and to search. She was the exceptional patient who triggered in me a desire to be a better therapist.

In the final chapter of this book we describe Vicky Clement Jones, a cancer patient who, in her own way, became an exceptional patient and triggered in Maurice Slevin, her doctor, and in all the people around her, a new approach to cancer patients. Reading this, one may ask oneself, "Can I become this exceptional creative patient?" The answer is in the trying. The use of the model of crisis was suggested earlier as a way of dealing with the "cancer situation". The three aspects of crisis are: lack of information, lack of support and lack of options. We discussed the two aspects of information and support, and tried to focus on the problems they each present for the person at the time of crisis. The lack of options, especially when faced with cancer, seems to be the biggest obstacle. Naturally, we assume an option means a solution and a solution to cancer is a cure. So what can one make of new options, if they are not related to cure?

## FINDING NEW OPTIONS

What crisis does to a person is not related only to the original event, but to a general feeling of hopelessness. Life without hope and choices is not life. Whether one is dealing with cancer, bereavement or separation, what we mean by "new options" is getting back into the driver's seat of one's own life. One of the questions which creates an impasse is, "What good can this or that do for my cancer?" New options are for the person, not necessarily for the cancer. When the person with the cancer moves on, there is no telling what he or she can discover in themselves. The human potential movement, influencing much of our contemporary thought, tells us that very little of our potential is used in normal life. That means we possess in ourselves much more energy, imagination, hope, talent and love than we usually use. The big question, of course, is, how can we put into use these stored treasures? Again, three main sources are mentioned as triggers: other people, accidental insights from books, groups, films and so on, but, more than those, the events of life itself. Cancer is an occurrence that triggers a general enlisting of resources. The threat it carries can be a stimulant to wake up and use a whole lot more of ourselves for life. The new options can be stimuli for better relationships, a different lifestyle, new beliefs or a greater degree of creativity. Faced with cancer, the question is not what options one chooses, but rather the fact one can and should choose. The freedom to recognise one has new possibilities is already a change. While the realisation of cancer creates a sense of loss of some options in life, the new freedom from fear gives birth to new potentials.

Cancer freedom may sound to many like a rather cynical combination of words. I would not have dared to use those words if I was not quoting directly from many cancer patients. It may well be that most people with cancer experience more anxiety and fear than freedom and new creativities. Any crisis is a dramatic change in life. One may be stuck in the middle of the drama and put all one's efforts into surviving it, but there are also other possibilities. Every dramatic change in life may produce new options triggering more potential. We all have unlived life within us. In Michelangelo's words, "This rock has in it an angel that wants to come out." But in sculpture, as in life, one has to hammer in order to release the angel.

Cancer victimises, but such persons can, by refusing to be passive victims, turn into heroes by trying to use their fight and spirit to gain knowledge, support and create new possibilities for themselves and others.

This chapter has tried to suggest a way of thinking. We were aware of the spontaneous questions that may arise in the readers' minds and have responded to rather grandiose concepts such as freedom, heroism and turning the tide. Since both authors of this book are practitioners, it is natural we will follow our ideas with more concrete examples in the following chapters.

# Chapter 2

# The weekend seminar

It is Friday night, in Oxford. The Conference Room on the second floor of Hopcroft's Holt Hotel is being used for the first time; we are launching it. All fresh, this spacious square room, with bright walls, soft carpeting and inviting chairs, looks over the English garden. During the afternoon our students, eleven couples, have arrived at this elegant old inn on the main road. As someone commented, "It looks like a weekend in the country with cocktails at 6.00 p.m." The young receptionist remarked, "Oh dear, is this the cancer group? Gosh, they don't look it." So we have already started to improve negative images surrounding cancer.

We meet for cocktails, our first encounter: twelve couples, patients and supporters and us, Maurice and Nira, Hedy Wax our administrator and Hilary Plant our senior oncology nurse.

Cocktails at 6.00 p.m. One can see the people wondering: "What are we doing here?" "How can this be a step in helping us deal with cancer?" One glance at the list of names and addresses, one look at the people, reveals a kaleidoscope of society in England today.

Janet and Gerry were young, sporty, she an American living in England, he a businessman. Both travelled constantly between London and New York, having been in many groups before this one. Veterans! In a corner of the room, a couple still by themselves. He in his early fifties, she a little younger. Margaret is a housewife and mother, Tom a leader of the Welsh miners. He has rarely left Wales. This weekend is an event in itself. Gretchen and Anton came to the seminar from Zurich; elegant, affluent, a lawyer and his wife. She was a housewife and hostess until she developed cancer and became a mountain climber. John and Harry, two male friends, are talking to Mave and her daughter Vera. Mave is from Cyprus, but her daughter is very English. Michael and Beverley: he is a lay preacher and accountant, she a teacher and active church volunteer. Ruth and Trevor: she is the patient, of Indian origin and he is a bus driver. They have never before participated in a group. Sandra and Barbara, friends, both are self-employed, one is an architect, the other owns a market garden. Ellen and Christopher, a middle-aged couple: she is talkative and surprisingly youthful, he, a successful journalist, is the patient. Graham and Jane: he is an optician, candid and confident, she is the patient, intense and very withdrawn. Peter and Rose: he is a businessman, she his part-time helper, the patient – the quietest couple.

A range of people of different ages, origins and socioeconomic status, but they have a common denominator. Not only do they share a diagnosis of cancer, they are all interested in an active struggle, ready to change and adapt, eager to learn and lucky enough to have at least one person in the world to call a friend or supporter.

Over the next one and a half days we all participated in discussions, presentations and encounters, part of a process leading to a change in perspectives about cancer. Our goals included: imparting information to the participants and encouraging them in their search for further information; stimulating the skills of self-support and being able to accept the support of others; exploring new ways of relating to wellbeing and new options for self-help; strengthening existing relationships; and reevaluating their present situations in a supportive atmosphere.

In the following chapter we have recorded a range of voices. The themes arose spontaneously from within the flexible framework of the seminars. We have attempted to capture the spirit of the discussions, concentrating on the dominant themes that emerged.

This verbatim has been put together from several seminars. The people are real, the stories are authentic. As the weekends developed, more and more people came for a second time and third time. The mix of people ranged not only between young and old, newly diagnosed and "chronic patients", but also supporters who became bereaved – and people who can be regarded as cured. People like Gretchen, the Swiss mountain climber, came several times to encourage others to believe cancer can mean a new freedom.

To maintain clarity, we have divided the discussions into short sections under thematic subheadings. We hope our experience and the insights acquired will encourage patients and supporters to develop a positive attitude towards facing cancer and to suggest it is possible to live a richer and more fulfilling life after diagnosis of cancer.

## DAY ONE

## Control

*Beverley:* Until I developed cancer I had always been very much in control, at least most of the time. I helped others, who were disabled, to cope with their lives, so when I was diagnosed it came as a shock to find I was not in a position to control anything, myself or anybody else. What I am hoping to gain from this weekend is to learn how to control the situations I am encountering at the moment.

*Barbara:* I am fairly new to this. My cancer was diagnosed about 6 weeks ago and I am in the middle of treatment. Similarly to Beverley, one thing that struck me at the beginning and which is still with me is suddenly not being in control of my life any more. I have always been someone who has absolute control over what I was doing, both for myself and other people. I just can't lead a normal life at the moment.

*Maurice:* What you have both described is very common among cancer patients and one of the ways cancer differs from many other illnesses. It appears we have much less influence over cancer and less understanding than of, say, heart disease. If you have angina, a pain in the chest which comes on when you are exercising, we know it is caused by a narrowing of blood vessels to the heart and the reason why you have the pain when you are exercising is your heart has to work harder and so it needs more oxygen. The blood vessels have narrowed, so it's not possible for extra blood to get to the heart and this causes pain. The positive thing about this pain is that you know when your angina is out of control as you will get chest pain after walking a certain distance. On the other hand, if your angina were controlled, you would notice you were able to walk quite far without difficulty and without getting chest pain.

With cancer, you feel well, go about your everyday life and suddenly develop a minor cough, a mild pain, or perhaps cough up a small amount of blood or find you are constipated. You're not particularly worried, but you go to the doctor. He investigates and the tests prove you have cancer. Suddenly it dawns on you, you have actually had this for quite a while. You have been leading a normal life, feeling quite happy, yet this cancer has been growing inside you, without any indication, in a suspicious and dishonest way. It has caused few or no symptoms and feels much more out of control than other illnesses where there is a relationship between the disease and the symptoms. You then go into hospital to see a range of specialists and are faced with investigations and treatment, some of which are quite unpleasant and you seem to have no control. You, of course, do have the ultimate control. You could refuse to have treatment, but most people in this situation are frightened and will do anything to make themselves better, so this is not a real option. These experts cannot give you definite answers about what caused the cancer, why it happened to you and cannot guarantee the results of treatment. So even they seem not to have control over the disease. You become part of the hospital system where you have clinic clerks, nurses, doctors, receptionists, social workers, telling you what to do. You are somebody who has previously controlled every aspect of life, and often the lives of many other people too, suddenly finding you're like a child again; you can no longer make your own decisions. The whole concept of running your own life your way and being in control of what happens changes overnight.

One of the main functions of this weekend is to help you to use your own resources to get back control of your lives, which you may feel has been lost. This doesn't apply only to the patients, but also to the relatives and friends supporting the patient and deeply involved in what is happening. Supporters are also thrown out of their routine and depend on others to tell them what to do.

*Nira:* Being a therapist for many years I often find myself with people struggling throughout their lives to be in control and who, all the time, have a sense of lack of control, a feeling of helplessness, a catastrophic anticipation of being found out and ridiculed. In a way we all share this anxiety and need to remind ourselves we're never really out of control. Even when we're asleep we don't actually fall out of bed. We sense we are at the edge of the bed and roll back.

In times of crisis, and a cancer diagnosis is a case in point, this is not just an anxiety, it is a reality. What is it about being diagnosed as having cancer that causes an instant lack of control? There are a number of issues that strike you upon being diagnosed, or perhaps only after you have recovered from the initial shock. There are at least four different stages, although obviously to different people they may come at different times and some people will only experience some or maybe none of these stages. First, as Maurice said, there's the realisation of a process that has been developing for some time in your body without you being aware of it, not to mention being able to control it. Your body at that point becomes a mystery. You realise that your personal style of controlling your body has failed you. Or if you never put much attention into your body until now, you realise that it is an existent entity, an autonomous being and right now it is dominant. From this minute on there is a separation of mind and matter, you are bound to rely on mind and spirit as matter seems out of control. I can think of the wife of a patient I saw recently who said to me that once her husband had been diagnosed as having cancer, the first thing they said to themselves was, "Well from now on it clearly has to be a case of mind over matter." The second issue that is a problem for many people is this question of other people, mainly doctors and nurses, but many other people also, including fellow patients, who form a cortège that starts to overtake your life. You realise that while you aren't controlling what's happening in your body, or what will happen, these other people are trying to do so. I call this the so-called invasion of the experts. Your life up to this point, although probably supported at times by experts, mostly took your own expertise to survive and guide you. But now survival depends on them and all these people have access to your body, your life and your future. So you are faced with your own private cancer, your own private body, but it is now no longer private, because of your tumour or growth, better known as cancer, or the big C or the disease whose name is not pronounced. You are struck by the myths of cancer, mainly that cancer is always fatal, no matter what "they" do. This feeling, however incorrect, is based on previous knowledge from people whom you knew that have died of cancer and it is very powerful. Your main resources in fighting your battle are the doctors, but most of them are anonymous to you in the same way that you are anonymous to them.

They may appear to be inaccessible; so are the facts and names and things that you don't understand, but at the back of your mind you feel that no matter how important they look, they, too, may be helpless to fight and conquer the big C. Everyone knows that patients still die of cancer, so their lack of control is known to you, you feel that their secret is out in spite of their manoeuvres. Later you'll have to decide deliberately to trust them, since they are in the front line and they are a great part of your strength, but for many people this will take time. Another difficulty that many people find is the almost total lack of partnership in treating your cancer. You are not asked to do anything to help, to work harder, to give up comfort, to economise, no skill whatever that in the past has been crucial to the solving of any problem is offered to you. That is interpreted as meaning only one thing, that no matter what you do or how skilful, or how disciplined or obedient you are, your cancer has nothing to do with you, only with others' skills. You are not asked to do anything. This is not only different to any other problem, but also to most other illnesses, which are always treated with the patient's collaboration. This message reads loud and clear: there is absolutely nothing that you can do. When all these things happen to you more or less at the same time, you cannot avoid a real sense of lack of control. This weekend is a step in the direction of helping you regain your sense of control and changing your attitude to these issues.

In order to gain control, I'd like to describe what it is that gives us a sense of control over ourselves and our lives. I'll only mention here some of the characteristics of the sense of control that are relevant to this issue. One is a connection between cause and effect. This is often very difficult with cancer because in many instances this is not known even by the experts, yet there still is information about how cancer arises and what goes wrong to allow it to happen. It is essential that you understand what is taking place, why first tests and treatments are being suggested, and are able to use this information in order to plan. You must also feel that you are able to rely on your skills, knowledge, hard work, willpower and support to help you overcome this problem. In the end we have to accept the structure in which we live, to respect expertise and to understand the different hierarchies around us. All this put together forms a freedom of choice: even though most of the time we can only choose from the available options, still there is freedom.

### Automatic pilot

*Barbara:* I feel apart from all the other people here; I haven't really got any positive ideas in my mind. I said earlier that I felt I wasn't in control of my life any more, but listening to other people here. I also find that I don't appear to have a positive attitude. I'm just letting the treatment wash over me at the moment, I realise that I put myself completely and utterly in the hands of the doctors and, although I thought positively about the end result of the treatment, I don't know quite what to expect of it. I can't lead a normal life at the moment, so I can't just pick up the threads, but in my mind I don't know how much I'm giving in to it.

*Nira:* I want to relate to what Barbara has said. I will try and quote her. She said that she just goes step by step, she does what the doctors tell her, she takes the treatment and later tries to think what she should be doing. Now this technique is called searching for the automatic pilot. You may all be familiar with the concept of automatic pilot. An automatic pilot in a plane is turned on and guides the plane having all the information about where to go. In life we often switch to automatic pilot. We use a large storage of previous experience, information and previous guidance. This is not just being automatic, it means using automatically previous knowledge and experience. Now even the sophisticated automatic pilot can only choose options and solutions that are programmed into it. It means that when we are on automatic pilot we have to trust our previous experience and knowledge and we cannot invent new things in this situation. Under stress or at times of crisis when decisions are very difficult, we are afraid that they are critical, and we are very afraid of making a mistake, so it is good instinctive behaviour to switch to automatic pilot. "Just do what I did in the past as it worked for me." Just rest for the meantime and don't try to find new solutions, don't work hard and regret a decision, just use what helped me in the past. It seems that what Barbara has said may be of relevance to many of you, who at times, especially perhaps after a major shock like the diagnosis of cancer, switch to automatic pilot.

*Maurice:* As Nira says, what Barbara describes here as just carrying on and not, in her words, "developing a fighting spirit" is, in fact, a very useful and healthy way of coping with this information at this point. Many people (I am sure many of you here have experienced this), when they are first diagnosed as having cancer, find it difficult to do just what she has done, to switch on to automatic pilot. This is because when they search for a previous response, when they try to find the stored information which enabled them to turn to automatic pilot, they find that that response does not exist. They then get stuck in a situation where they are unable to make new decisions because they are not yet ready to do so, and also unable to fall back on an automatic pilot. This provokes a feeling of panic and is one of the components of being in a crisis.

Many people with cancer talk somewhat paradoxically about how the cancer has in some ways changed their lives for the better. Cancer is often a disease of mid-life, or of older people, and at this time many people are living their lives mostly on automatic pilot. This is the more negative aspect of using your automatic pilot. People find that life carries on in the same way that it always has and that there's no reason to try new things. They fear exchanging the feeling of comfort which comes of doing things in the same old way as before for the potential excitement and stimulation. Sometimes it requires an illness like cancer to push people off course and force them to stop living their life completely in automatic pilot. When this happens they may suddenly start seeing life from a new perspective and feel that new perspective to be one of the positive effects of having this illness.

## The wisdom of the desert

*Janet:* My doctor kept mis-diagnosing me, telling me there was probably something wrong with my head rather than in my chest. Eventually I was getting sicker and sicker and the doctor did a chest X-ray and found a lump in my chest. I then had an operation and I was diagnosed as having Hodgkin's disease. It was diagnosed in the United States and I decided not to go back to England for the treatment. When I was first diagnosed I asked the oncologist what I could do for myself. He said he didn't believe in any of that; that he could get me better. He told me they can do a lot for Hodgkin's disease and then, as you said earlier, I went more or less on automatic pilot. I just committed myself to chemotherapy and didn't think very much about it at all. But then I was getting very depressed, I was always very pessimistic about my treatment. I couldn't see anything positive coming out of it at all. He suggested I went to a psychiatrist and I did. This was very helpful; it was more psychotherapy than psychoanalysis. At that time I had a bit more free time and I decided to read about Hodgkin's disease. I suppose I was coming out of the automatic-pilot stage and wanting to get some more control. I would pick up one or two pamphlets which were always in the doctor's office and things like that. They were very depressing to read as they always talked about 5-years' survival rate and I wished they had come up with some other way of presenting the statistics. I spoke to my oncologist in New York about getting involved in a group but he was very much against it, saying that individual therapy is fine, but right now he didn't feel I needed to be dealing with the emotions of other people and that therapy in a group with some people who were worse than me would make me more depressed. However, I did go and see a group without his approval and I found that quite helpful.

Coming back to England I tried to find a psychiatrist here and tried two or three before I found one that I liked. Along the way I came across a very interesting man who was very much involved in alternative therapy for cancer, which was very enlightening, but I always questioned his basic premiss that you could affect the outcome of the illness with these alternative treatments. I also didn't like the idea suggested by the alternative therapist that I had something to do with the onset of the cancer and was therefore to blame for it. I left this therapist because of our basic differences. I continued to do a lot more reading about Hodgkin's disease and delved into some of the professional writing about it just to learn more and more about it, about the drugs and about what the disease was. Once I settled down I began to exercise and that made a very big difference, it made me feel that my life was coming together again. I still have a lot of trouble trying to ignore the fears and at times I am totally consumed by them and there are also times when they go away. One of these times was when we went to the mountains. The other time was when we were in the hills on holiday. It was incredible how both times, when we were very active and doing things, one of them was skiing and the other was just swimming and sightseeing, how this helped me to put things into perspective. There were times when I was able to ignore the fears and my obsession with cancer and rise above it somehow to gain a little more control. I don't know if it was getting out of the city and a bit closer to nature or something, or closer to the elements, but it made a tremendous difference. When I got back to London I started swimming and taking exercise and that has been very helpful to me.

*Gretchen:* I was a patient with breast cancer two years ago. I never had a mastectomy, but I had an operation to remove the lump and then had radiotherapy. Before developing cancer and having this treatment, I was a very good housewife and a mother. I was always willing for anybody to come home and have dinner. I used to cook and if they came back late and spoilt the meal that I had cooked, I was always very nice about it. My husband loves golf and I'd trot along every weekend and play golf although I hated it. I mean I would complain; it wasn't that I didn't ever tell him I didn't like it, but although I complained I still went along. Suddenly last summer after radiotherapy, I felt very angry. The first thing I started doing, I suddenly started climbing mountains. Rock climbing. This is a very strange thing to do because I suffer from vertigo, but it was excellent. It was the right way because it taught me one thing. With rock climbing, you have to stay in the present. Only the next step is important, not the rest of the way to the top of the mountain. If I look down I get vertigo, so I just look at the next grip and I also say to God, "I dare you to shake me off this rock." But my husband's had a hard time with all this and my children have had a hard time. He doesn't like going to opera or theatre and suddenly I started going to them and really liked them. It seems that I am being very good to myself, but I am giving my family a hard time. I also must say that I felt suddenly very isolated and alone in this. On the one hand, I enjoy life much more. I almost had the feeling that I got cancer (I don't know if this is right or wrong) because I was paying too much attention to what I should do from the outside and to what I was expected to do. Now I am much better to myself and I have my new-found courage, but it also scares me.

**Being alone**

*Nira:* You talk about how it felt exciting but also frightening. With your new-found courage you felt alone. You describe not loneliness, but being alone for better or worse. I feel I have the courage to do things, but it scares me. Now this feeling of being alone has nothing to do with how many people you have around you. Many times it is very frustrating for family members and friends when they've put a lot of effort into supporting you and you still say that you feel alone or lonely and your husband or wife or sister says, "But I've been here every day for the last year." They feel insulted and frustrated. It has nothing to do with what they are trying to do for the person, it's simply that being under the stress of crisis makes an old truth even more poignant. We are alone, not that people don't love us, but there's a certain "aloneness" in the human condition for better or for worse. Unless we are under the stress of crisis, we don't think about it every day; we are together with the family and at work, but once something like this really hits us, the first thing we experience is, "I'm alone." I can sit with you and hold your hand if you suffer pain. Maybe I can help you a little just with sympathy, but you still suffer the pain. I don't. Sometimes with cancer, especially in a marriage, there may be a degree of overprotection. Your partner may say "we both have it", but that is not true; only one of you has the cancer. I can do the best I can for you, but you have the cancer and you have to face being alone. Being alone has a frightening part, but it also has enormous power and we should not deny it altogether, for then we also deny our power. It's frightening because once you accept that you're alone and you take responsibility for yourself, it feels like you're out of the clan, that you don't have everyone else's support. There is also a slight fear of rejection. "If I don't need them, perhaps they don't need me." But the power comes from being able to do for yourself the things that you believe to be right for you. So you suddenly realise, "I can do it, I can climb mountains, I can go on my own to the theatre. Even though I've never been before, all of a sudden not only can I go, but I can also enjoy it." There is no reason why you could not have done it before. The potential to do it was always there. Exercise, mountain climbing, enjoying looking at life differently, you do it all now because you have cancer, but it's also a bit scary, especially because of the way it affects your relationship with your husband and with your children. We are all frightened of change.

Both Gretchen and Janet have mentioned something else. Janet talked about going for walks in the hills, finding out about the value of exercise; Gretchen about climbing mountains, going to the theatre for the first time on her own. What have these got to do with cancer? What has mountain climbing got to do with trying to overcome a crisis of this sort? I'd like to use a quote here from Reverend Johnson, who was head of Gethsemane Church in Jerusalem for many years, in his paper entitled "The wisdom of the desert". He discusses the need to get away from a pressing problem, to go to the desert whether actually, or symbolically, to do other things, to gain control of something, no matter what. The desert is a place which contains no greenery, no water, no actions, no tools to overcome any hardship. There is no life; it is, in fact, a sort of vacuum. Instead of meditating on the uncontrollable, get away, clear your mind, behave "as if" you are not busy with your problem. "As if" means not to deny, not to defy, but just to clear your mind. In all that time a solution is forming within you. The desert will bring enlightenment and a solution will come. To rephrase that, one rarely finds a solution to a problem at the level of the problem.

*Maurice:* It is clear that climbing mountains, exercising and going to the theatre are not solving the problem of cancer. They're certainly not a solution at that level. But somehow, for both Janet and Gretchen, by doing these things there was a solution to the impasse that they were facing. I'm not saying that it is never the right thing to do to tackle the problem directly. Initially Janet did exactly that by trying to see different doctors, reading about the cancer and so on, but when a problem cannot be resolved, maybe the only way to solve it is to "go to the desert".


## DAY TWO

### Past, present, future

*Trevor:* Over the past year I've had a period of absolute uncertainty. My wife has had a series of operations and treatments and no time to recover from the surgery before the next one has happened. The point hasn't yet been reached when I can begin to think of what new direction to go in. Up till now all I could keep up with were the pure mechanics of maintenance and all I can think of for the moment is getting back to something more or less like the way we used to live. Ruth's cancer has been a major disruption in our lives and all I can think of is trying to get things back to the way they were.

*Nira:* I'd like to relate to the last point. We all know there are three times in life, the past, the present and the future. In crisis there is only one time; the past. The future is just obscure and the present is very difficult. We have only one hope and that is that things will be the way they used to be, the way they were the moment before the situation occurred. Everything in the past seems better than what is happening now, so we think of the past. This will come up many times on the weekend and many of you have already expressed it in one way or another, being in the past, bringing things back to normal and similar phrases. Why is the future so obscure? It is because the present is so intense and so difficult. To talk about next week seems a long way away. The future is not next year, the future is the next 24 hours. So when you are in crisis time takes on a totally different dimension. The question is: how am I going to survive the crisis over the next 24 hours? The only thing that counts is what we are going to do today. The wish to go back to the past is, of course, unrealistic. Not only is it impossible to go back in time to the same situation, but as people we cannot undo what has been done. When someone recovers from cancer they are not the same as before they had cancer because they have been through that experience.

### Living with advanced cancer

*Maurice:* When we talk about changing perspectives, we simply mean changing our attitude or our thoughts about having cancer. Now a very reasonable response would be, "Well, what good's that going to be?" The fact of the matter is that at the moment I have got cancer and simply changing my thoughts about it is not going to make it go away. That of course is absolutely true, but changing the way you view cancer can completely alter your feelings about it and, as a result of that, your quality of life. I would like to use a very simple example quoted in a book by an American psychiatrist named Gerald Jampolsky to illustrate this point. You go into a restaurant, an expensive restaurant, and order a meal. Despite paying a lot of money, the service is awful. The waitress looks dishevelled, she is inattentive, inconsiderate and sometimes rude. On one occasion she spilt the soup on the table and didn't even apologise. By the end of the evening you are in a bad mood, you have not enjoyed your meal, you call the manager over and complain and do not leave a tip. You feel angry that this evening you had looked forward to has been spoilt.

Let's envisage exactly the same situation but, just before you sat down, the friend you were with whispered in your ear that the waitress has just lost her husband and has a young child at home who is sick, whom she has left with a neighbour because she cannot afford not to go to work. She feels depressed and alone and is worried sick about her child. You would now view this situation entirely differently, despite the waitress's lack of consideration and inattention; you would smile at her warmly, thank her for her help when she brought you the food, and do your best to be encouraging to her. At the end of the evening you would leave an extra large tip, and would leave the restaurant feeling sorry for her, but feeling quite good in yourself because you know that you gave her a degree of comfort from the way you behaved towards her. This information about the waitress would have added another dimension to your evening which you would have enjoyed, despite the difficulties with the service. This simple story illustrates how your attitude can dramatically influence your feelings.

Professor Kenneth Calman wrote an article in the *Journal of Medical Ethics* about quality of life as a cancer patient (Calman 1984). This article could easily have been entitled, "How does one find happiness?" or something similar. He put forward a very simple proposition that one's quality of life or happiness is just the difference between what you have and what you expect. The greater this gap the less your "quality of life" or the less your happiness and the smaller the gap the closer you will be to what you want. This is a very important and optimistic hypothesis, because very often in life it is difficult to change what we have, especially if a situation is created by something which is beyond our control, such as a physical illness. What we can always change is our expectations and we all do that all the time. A good example that we all have experienced is when we go to the theatre, or go to dinner, and we are not really looking forward to being with those people, or the play doesn't sound like one which we are going to enjoy. Don't we often come back from an evening like that saying, "I had a great time and it was much better than I expected." We know this so well, that when someone starts to tell us about how good a play is, we sometimes stop them and say, "Don't tell me about it; you will build my expectations up too high and I'm now going to find it disappointing."

When we become ill, part of our natural means of coping is to adjust our expectations to some extent. For example, someone who is ill in bed for a long time will get tremendous satisfaction and pleasure out of being able to walk round the garden for the first time for a long while. Having had an operation and not being able to eat for 2 weeks, the pleasure of that first mouthful is better than a gourmet meal in the best restaurant. This all relates to the fact that we had got used to being in bed and not being able to eat. Our expectations were very low and, as a result, very simple things were able to give us great pleasure and happiness. It is my experience that those patients with cancer, for that matter those people in life who are able to get the most pleasure, are those who are able always to adjust their expectations so that the gap between what they have and their expectations is always narrow. That is something which is available to all of us all the time. A patient of mine, Vicky Clement Jones, who was also a doctor, and who started the Cancer Information Service, BACUP, always used to amaze everyone with how she seemed to get such a great pleasure out of life, despite difficulties which would have seemed overwhelming to other people. Her secret was the ability continually to adjust her horizons and expectations so that she always had things to look forward to and had the satisfaction of achieving her aims and expectations, no matter how limited her physical capability.

*Janet:* I feel almost guilty saying this, but cancer can have a good side too. I've never been as generally happy as I am now. Some moments in nature and my general feeling of loving life are somehow much more important now. The colours are more intense, everything is more beautiful and I wouldn't miss it for anything in the world. The strange thing is that I never noticed so many things before I was diagnosed as having cancer. At first I thought that I should not feel like that. Then I remembered some stories of soldiers just before they went into battle, stories about how they lived much more intensely. I now live much more consciously and intensely and I find beauty in much more than I used to.

*Beverley:* I'd like to say something about this as well. I had just the same feelings after my treatment when I was feeling well again. I just got so much more out of simple things which I didn't even notice before. I felt that it would have been a pity to miss the opportunity of knowing what I now know and in some ways I would not have wanted to have missed this experience. I know that sounds very strange after what I've said earlier, but it's a bizarre feeling that I really do have. In fact, now that I'm feeling well again and have been for some time, I'll start drifting back into normality and sometimes I have to stop myself and say, "Hey, you're going back to what you were like before." I'm scared sometimes that I'll lose the new perspective I've gained in the past few months.

*Trevor:* When Ruth first got ill she felt that she needed to tidy up her life and organise everything so that she was prepared for anything that might happen. Well, I share an office with a very neat and organised person and I am exactly opposite, so it is very irritating to him. For me sorting out my life, trying to organise it, tidying my drawers, making my will and getting my life into a very tidy state, would make me feel that it was the end of life for me. I depend on the irritation of disorganised things around me to keep me going.

*Janet:* I think there is a distinction between tidying and coming to terms with cancer. I can remember the panic when I was first diagnosed that there were so many things that were unfinished. I was in the middle of moving into a new house, and all sorts of things needed to be done. I panicked, I needed to do these things and get them sorted out. I had the feeling I've got to take the time now to sort things out. I got a lot of enjoyment doing it, but there was a negative aspect to it, what I called a black edge, the feeling that I'm doing all this for the last time. Maybe, I won't ever be able to do it again. For some reason, thank goodness, it has now gone. I find it much easier to be conscious that these things might end, but just enjoy them for what they are for the moment. I think you sometimes need to do some tidying, but that's not all there is to it.

*Maurice:* Do you know what made the edge go away? What was different in the way you saw life then, and the way you see life now?

*Janet:* I think time has helped, it's been nearly 18 months. Initially I found it very difficult when people suggested to me that I should take each day at a time, I felt I wanted to get back to what life was like in the past, come back to that blissfully ignorant state when I didn't ever think I was going to die, or at least that I'd live till old age. You just assume you're going to go on and you never think about death. I resented terribly people saying that I should strive to take each day at a time because that was acknowledging that there might not be too many tomorrows. I really resented that approach to me. I didn't want to take each day at a time, I wanted to go back to being able to assume that life would continue. It was a dilemma for me that I couldn't go back to the ignorance that I had before. I think what took the black edge out of what I was doing was simply time itself. I now do live day by day, but I do it without thinking that I'm living one day at a time; but it was having to do it consciously that felt difficult.

*Beverley:* I think taking each day at a time in my experience doesn't mean that today is all you have, but that today is here to be made the most of. In the past I had the luxury of feeling that today didn't matter because I had lots of tomorrows, that was a luxury, but it also had negative aspects. One of the big things that has happened to me since having cancer is that I appreciate today, I appreciate the present rather than always thinking that good things are going to happen in the future.

*Maurice:* You're seeing this concept of "living each day at a time" from a different perspective. Janet is talking about the fact that living each day at a time implies that she hasn't got too many days left and

Beverley is saying that she now sees life in a different perspective and wants to get more value out of each day, irrespective of whether she has a short time to live or is going to live to old age. This is another example of how important perspective is. The same issue for two different people can evoke very different feelings, in fact opposite feelings. I think what Janet says brings up important issues about the question of how people feel when they believe that their life is limited to a fixed period of time. In fantasy terms we all really have difficulty coming to terms with the fact that we are going to die even though we all know it will happen at some time. It's often said that that's the only real certainty in life. We don't, however, live every day of our lives taking that fact into account. We don't plan a holiday or career, to take into account the fact that whatever we do we will eventually die. John Harris in his book, *The Value of Life* (Harris 0000), talks about how essential it is for us to believe that life is potentially unlimited. Once we put a fixed time limit on the duration of life, it may discolour and devalue that time that we actually do have left. You often hear of patients recounting how their doctor said they had 6 months or a year or 3 years to live. You usually hear people talking about this at a cocktail party 10 years later, when they tell you they send an annual Christmas card to their doctor to remind him that they are still here. For many people, being given such information is tantamount to having a death sentence pronounced and this small piece of information can substantially interfere with their quality of life. I think it is almost always a mistake for a doctor to give this information. It is well known that doctors cannot make such predictions and that it is always uncertain how long an individual patient is going to live. Statistics are useful for doctors to compare different sorts of treatment because they tell you how long an average patient is going to live. What they don't do is tell you anything about the individual patient you encounter the next day in the clinic. That patient could die in a very short while or could live a normal life expectancy and no doctor, however clever, can actually predict that accurately. I think the comment that Janet makes is relevant to many people who feel that they still want potentially to regard their lives as being of indefinite length in exactly the same way as somebody who doesn't have cancer. Clearly they have to take into account that it might be much shorter and to plan for that, but then to try and go on living life without having to consider how long they've got to live before carrying out any particular task. If you do this it makes it very difficult to do anything in a carefree and lighthearted way, without weighing up whether it's appropriate in terms of the time you've got left.

*Margaret:* I've been listening to everything that people have been saying about having a positive attitude and fighting spirit and changing perspective and so on. I know this sounds, in a way, defeatist and negative, and I'm really scared of saying it because I feel that I might be being harmful to Tom. It does worry me to think that he's not feeling well at the moment and he's going to put all this effort and time into trying to do these things and feeling positive. I know that he's going to work very hard at it and I know that I'll help him, but I feel that if in the end he dies anyway, then wouldn't it have been just better for him to have an easy time, and to relax and not take on all these new pressures, just enjoy life rather than try all these new things? Sometimes I feel that maybe it is all a waste of time anyway, is it worth all this bothering unless you know for certain it's going to help?

*Maurice:* It's not so much a case of whether or not we'll succeed in getting over the cancer, it's not so much whether or not in the end, you actually do or do not die of cancer, because, finally, all of us are obviously going to die. None of us knows when that will be. None of us knows whether it will be a long or a short time. But it's something that nobody can evade; we cannot avoid death as part of life. If you live long enough your grandparents will die, if you live longer, your parents will die, if you live longer, your friends and your spouse will die, if you live longer it's your children that will die and if you live long enough even your grandchildren will die. You reach a point at which it is part of life. The whole thing about being here on this weekend is that people want to do something for themselves, and to be involved in the fight against cancer for themselves. Now if you get involved in the fight and if, in the end, the cancer progresses, ultimately you still die of cancer, does that mean that being involved in the fight was a complete waste of time? Does it mean you tried and failed? If that is so then the whole of life is a failure, because the end of all life is death. Therefore, what is the point of us being here in the first place, going through all these struggles when we're going to die anyway? Not only are we going to die, but everything else we do, all the children we produce, everything they produce, are also going to die. So if death is seen as a failure, then there is no point in living. Having cancer just makes you focus on life and death. You're always faced with the possibility of death; with cancer things suddenly become more acute. But it is not whether you live or whether you die, whether you get over the cancer or whether you don't get over the cancer in the end. What matters is that you're involved in the struggle. That you are involved in the attempt, in the process of fighting, of trying to do something for yourself to help yourself. So getting involved in relaxation or exercise or any of the other things we suggest, some of them, all of them, or none of them, changes your perspective and your belief, how you feel about what's happening to you, and that's what it is all about. There will come a time when all of us, maybe when we're 60, maybe when we're 70, maybe when we're 90, maybe even 120, have reached the point where we're going to have to die. And life has actually to come to some natural end. What matters is our perspective about that when the time comes, and when we're ready to die. There are many people who get cancer who would not even think about wanting to be involved in any way with "fighting cancer", dealing with it or taking control of themselves. They're happy to leave things up to their doctor and to fate and that is fine. Other people have a need to be involved with the fight and the purpose of these weekends is to help direct that process. If one thinks that life is going to be shorter, if it's going to be less than the average, the same criteria apply as they do to a normal lifespan. What matters is not whether you die or don't die; that's certain. What matters is what happens in the middle. This concept of doing something for yourself doesn't necessarily mean that you can help yourself to get rid of the cancer, but the actual process of doing it may make a big difference to your beliefs and your attitude and the way you think about things and what happens to you.

*Beverley:* I'm not sure if this is irrelevant, but last night after dinner we were talking about the fact that cancer gives you time to get accustomed to the fact that you may have to die and that is sometimes a frightening thing, but also it's quite reassuring. Last week there was a sermon in church which changed my mind about dying suddenly. In the past, whenever I heard of a sudden death like a heart attack or something like that, I'd say how marvellous for them and what a terrible shock for the family. Well, this wonderful man that we have in our church who gave the sermon said that it's all wrong to take that line because it is not marvellous for someone to go suddenly. He said the majority of us would rather have time to think about whatever we're going to, whatever our beliefs, and prepare ourselves to a certain extent.

*Maurice:* That's a very interesting comment. It certainly fits in with what I would feel for myself, but it's not what everyone would feel. Some people would undoubtedly want to die very quickly and suddenly, while others would prefer to have time to sort things out. I went to West Germany a few years ago to a conference on bereavement. We had a number of group workshops and in the group that I was in there were about thirty people. I was actually the only doctor, but there were social workers, teachers, nurses, who were all involved in one way or another with bereavement. As part of it we had an exercise, a sort of fantasy about how you would want to die yourself. You had to choose everything about your death, including where you die, how will it be, who'd be there and also what you died of. There were only two people in the group who actually worked full-time with cancer; one was myself and the other a psychotherapist who worked on a children's cancer ward. All the others were involved with bereavement in one way or another, but not specifically with cancer patients. The thing that interested me was that only two people in the group chose to die of cancer. One of them was me and the other was the psychotherapist who worked with cancer patients. None of the others chose cancer. Having said that, I would, of course, be quite selective about what sort of cancer I chose. Why is it that none of the other people chose to die of cancer? Most of them in fact chose to die very suddenly of a heart attack. I think a large part of it may be due to misconceptions people have about cancer, the feeling that people have that it's a prolonged and painful and awful death, something that anybody looking after a cancer patient knows simply isn't true for the great majority of patients. Many people don't have pain and those that do can almost always have it well controlled with modern medication. From my point of view I don't see it in such a negative context, perhaps because I am used to dealing with cancer patients and don't suffer from all the misconceptions that other people have. But I can actually see a lot of advantages, an advantage to having a chance to be able to come to terms with dying and with yourself, other people, to sort things out in your life over a period of time; to round off your life. After we had discussed it, several other people in the group were won over to the concept that knowing you're going to die, and having the opportunity to think about things, having some control over what is happening to you, and how you ended your life, had a lot of advantages.

*Beverley:* I've met a lot of old people in old people's homes. You see them slowly disintegrating, sometimes they disintegrate physically with their minds probably being alright, but unable to do anything. And other times they become quite senile. I've looked at them and thought, "This is all wrong. Life shouldn't be like this." And I've often thought even before I became ill that I'd rather have an illness like cancer where I'd be surrounded by people who care in one way or another if I am going to die, to do it with self-respect, not having lost control over my mind and being totally dependent on other people looking at me and feeling sorry for me.

**Loneliness versus being alone**

*Nira:* In this group, over this weekend, we have a non-representative sample of people, not only because the reason for coming here is that either you or the person you are supporting has cancer, but also because there is no-one here who is lonely. People have come as couples whether related as husbands and wives or as friends or as parents and children. Every person in this group has a supporter, and every supporter has someone to support, even we who are co-ordinating the seminar are supporting each other.

It may look as if there is only one thing that we are avoiding here, and that is being alone. Dealing with loneliness is one thing, and dealing with being alone is another. Very often we confuse the two, and regard both of them as positions which should be avoided.

Let's discuss being alone first. In this discussion we will very briefly look at the socialisation process that initially takes place during childhood and young adulthood and continues throughout life. Socialisation is our developmental process for finding our place amongst people and learning to interact in a meaningful way. We will use the blackboard just to draw graphically so it will be easier for the group.

The child is the centre of his circle-universe. The first circle of belonging within which he learns to interact is with one other person, usually his mother. The second circle is when his universe widens and he learns to interact with his second circle which will usually consist of the father and the rest of the family. This universe goes on widening for school, clubs, college, political parties and many more circles of belonging and interactions. All this time the child–person remains right at the centre, the only centre possible, of all these widening circles. In each circle he interacts with many or few other people, but he and he alone is the person that belongs to this family, this club, this political party, this neighbourhood, this clinic, this office, in that order and combination. It is also only he that has all the memories, associations, and so on. In other words, there is only one person who is at the centre of his universe, and, following this little illustration, there can be no other as no circle can have more than one centre. That person is me, only me, and me alone. This being alone is a reality, whether we like it or not, whether we run away from it or not, whether we are aware of it or not. We can choose to be afraid of it, deny it, or make peace with that universe. That is ME. My being alone, or rather my uniqueness, does not isolate me; it distinguishes me. Once I come to terms with my being alone, I am able to produce something unique be it in love, creation or the way I carry on. Awareness of my uniqueness, is my source of power.

Loneliness is a feeling that possesses us when we are not in touch with others actually or spiritually. Whether by force of circumstances or by self-isolation, inferiority, feelings of competitiveness or fear, if we are not in touch with others or even with one other person, then this agonising feeling of loneliness takes over. It is essential for us to distinguish being alone from loneliness because being alone is the fundamental characteristic of life itself. It will always be there and in many ways there is no point fighting it, rather we must learn to accept it and even like it. Being alone can turn out to be very positive, a strength, once we have come to terms with it. If you confuse loneliness and being alone you will spend your life in the frustrating attempt to drag another person to the centre of your circle to share it with you. This is something, which, in reality, is very difficult, if not impossible, to achieve. Growing up is differentiating love and closeness from being alone. When you are holding my hand it feels a great deal better, but my headache is still there and it is still my headache. However much you care for me, my headache and my cancer cannot be transferred to you. You can share my dreams, fantasies, skills and understandings. Sharing all these things with you creates another universe of two or more, but it is still composed of two people who are unique and alone. When a cancer patient says they feel alone and everyone around them, husbands, children and friends, look in dismay and horror and say, "How could you possibly feel alone? I've been there at your side the whole time" what they are referring to is the existential feeling of being alone. For many people the only time in life when they experience this feeling of being alone is when they face a crisis like cancer. Why is this? Because a lot of us spend much of our time doing things, setting goals and keeping active specifically so that we do not have this feeling. And it is when we are hit by something like cancer, that stops us in our tracks, that we are forced for the first time, perhaps, to come face to face with this absolute truth about life itself.

*Mave:* When you have an illness, you are very alone. You initially have to work through it yourself. For some months after I found I had cancer, I used to talk to myself and try to sort it out in my own mind. As I was driving around I was sort of having conversations with myself. In fact, I still do. At first I used to do it for about 4 hours a day and I used to think, you know, "I'm going crazy." I think it had a function really, I feel it was a way of sorting myself out. It was necessary and it was necessary for me to do it by myself, nobody else could really help me over that. I was unaware that anyone else has felt that.

*Harry:* I have too. When my wife left me, I did something I hadn't done for years, I got out my camping gear, my small tent, put it in my car and drove off to Exmoor with some walking boots, on my own. I did it because I needed to be alone. Because the pressures of everything were so great I thought, "I have to get away from everything and everyone I know and be on my own." I was also talking to myself in the car and I am sure that it was part of exorcising my fears and the stresses from my being. When I was alone in the country I met other people, I listened to music, I walked in the countryside of Exmoor on my own. When I came back I felt refreshed and much stronger. I never think that I am alone, but that is because of my religious feelings. It was a good thing, it was a gut feeling, that I had to do this, and it worked for me. I felt spiritually better. Physically I was better because I had fresh air and exercise, which I hadn't been getting because I had been neglecting myself. So I understand loneliness and being alone in terms of weakness and strength. "Lonely" seems to conjure up a feeling of being inept and not functioning as one should, but being alone feels like being strong and saying, "I don't need anyone for this period of time, I don't need anyone in fact, I need to be alone."

*John:* I am not sure that this is in the same context, but one of the things I like is going fishing. It is my way of getting away and being alone. Away from everything else, the family, and just totally, absolutely, relaxing. I am not really alone because obviously there are other things going on around me. You have the wildlife, the birds and everything else. But if I have a particular problem, something I need to sort out, I find it much easier if I can just go fishing and be on my own and just try to sort things out in my mind. It may not be in the same context as Harry was saying, but that's my way of being alone; not lonely in any sense of the word, just being on my own and being alone. Obviously from time to time I do meet other people when I go, but I sit there for hours on end, alone, and still enjoy myself and relax and come back feeling much better.

*Barbara:* I always associate being alone with loneliness, and I was always quite terrified of it, with the result that I have never been alone in my life. I always felt I needed someone else to enjoy things, that I couldn't see a nice film and enjoy it on my own. I have always felt that I have to be with someone. I always feared dying on my own. I felt I needed someone very close to me to be with me at the time, but more recently I have changed completely. I really need to be alone, especially since I had the cancer diagnosed. I found I just needed much more space to myself, going on a really long walk on my own and talking to myself. I started off feeling frustrated, angry and upset, and came back feeling completely different. This was an enormous experience for me, because I have always thought that being on my own meant being really miserable.

*Michael:* I think that another word that should be brought in is "solitude". I think solitude and being alone are two different concepts. Solitude is self-chosen isolation, coming to peace with yourself. When my wife was first seriously ill, I felt alone, but there was no-one who could really deeply and fully understand. That to me was being alone, whereas solitude is self-selected.

*Ruth:* Yes, I think of loneliness as being at home and being really lonely. But I have found that I have been in a crowd of people and been really lonely, which surprises me, because I thought if you were in a crowd you shouldn't be lonely. But I have felt really lonely being amongst the crowd. I always connect loneliness with being at home, but that is not true, it can affect you in exactly the same way when you are with people, and I have found that being alone is something I quite enjoy. When I am on my own I think about the people that care about me and do love me, so I know that they are still there, but I still enjoy my moments of being alone. Probably if I didn't have anybody else, those moments of being alone would be terrible. Because you have got other people who are really around you, you just need this time on your own.

*Janet:* Can you be alone with other people?

*Nira:* Many people in this room experience being alone all their lives, ever since their childhood.

*Barbara:* I find my priorities have changed. I find I am intolerant of simple conversations. I do not express this outwardly when I am with people, I listen, but switch off if I feel like switching off.

*Mave:* I can certainly identify with that; as a reaction to stress, there are times when you are just not there. I mean, I'm going through the motions, but there is an interior part of me that is sorting out something else at the same time. I'm talking, I'm communicating, I'm answering the question, but I'm not there. And it is something that happens. It is my reaction if there is something I need to sort out.

*Trevor:* I'd like to take it on from there. I haven't thought this through awfully well, but it can be very lonely to be with somebody, to be talking to somebody, and know they have left you behind. They've gone on, and it is my instinct to carry on and pretend it is not happening. I'm beginning to realise that sometimes I'm going to have to confront it, or certainly acknowledge it, and adjust, so I don't feel cut off.

*John:* I think I have difficulty feeling ready to open up in this group. I find it difficult to communicate. It's not a lack of will, it's more that I don't know what to communicate because I don't understand it myself.

*Nira:* Or is it because you don't believe that what you have to say is very important, and that unless you have something important to say, you will keep quiet? In that sense, one may never be ready.

*John:* I feel inhibited.

*Nira:* Yes, but once you start you become ready. There are certain things in life that you are not ready to do, but you do as you go along. The best example is to speak about the potential. We all know that we use a very small part of our potential. A psychologist once said that he didn't know anything more impotent than potential. He said "potential" is something you only know after it has happened. In retrospect. If someone achieves something you may say this person had the potential, but you know that in every first grade in school there are 30 or 40 geniuses. I mean they all have potential, but what happens later? Potential is not like a treasure deposited and then retrieved from a safe. Potential is more like the battery of a car. It recharges as you go. If you want to be ready, it never happens. If you don't start driving you don't go out at all. If you want to learn to speak up in groups or share your ideas, you cannot wait for yourself to be ready. This is a battery, where you speak to people and you get their reaction, and as you go on you learn, and refine your thoughts. The difficulty for many people in groups like this is, they say to themselves, "Look at all these smart people, at what they say." Nora spoke earlier about not talking and saying she felt "housewifeish". What that really means is that you are so ambitious that you feel unless you have got something really bright to say, you won't speak up, and what happens then is you stay lonely. So you need to learn to use your opportunities. Although this wasn't the reason most of you came to this group, this is an opportunity to speak up. Never mind if you have a hard time speaking up, this, in itself, is progress. In the next session you will say something more, simply because you have said something once.

*Barbara:* I'm not a lonely person, I don't suffer from loneliness. But once a week I like to be alone, if one can call it that. I go to an art class and when I am there I become so absorbed in what I am doing that I become alone. I am myself, doing my own thing. Not having to participate in conversation because everybody becomes their own selves, and just loses themselves in what they are doing. Is that what it is to be alone?

*Nira:* Yes. That's why it is not loneliness, it is nothing to do with the presence of people around us. It sometimes comes out as a problem in a family or relationship. When you have two people, and one has a need to be alone by going away fishing, or having a drink in the country or even in the house, the other person sometimes doesn't understand that. Because the other person doesn't have that need, he or she might interpret that as rejection, and that becomes important.

*John:* I experienced being alone among other people in my National Service a long time ago. I was sent abroad in the army with my friends. We went on the same boat and when, after a while, I was made a sergeant, I found I couldn't mix with them any more. It wasn't permissible. In fact I was ticked off more than once for trying to keep a foot in both camps. I was only 20. It took time for the penny to drop. I experience this now in management, I can't mix too much with the men; I have to keep myself apart to some degree. We can still talk and have a liaison, but it is limited. It is not a comradeship that exists when you are on the same level, such as when I first went into the army.

*Barbara:* I feel being alone can sometimes be forced on you. At times it becomes rather difficult to communicate with some of your friends. I find this because they are, in my eyes, living a superficial sort of life. I listen to them, but I am not really part of their conversation because what they are saying and talking about has got past me in a sense. That's happened since I got cancer.

## Survival

*Nira:* I'd like to talk about the concept of survival. The *Oxford English Dictionary* describes survival as "living longer than, or beyond the life of, another person". It is clear that although in every minute in life there are so many dangers, we only relate to "surviving" when there is an awareness of danger and when we need to make a conscious effort to overcome and live beyond that danger. That is why dealing with cancer requires, apart from treatment, a skill for survival.

While many believe that this is a special asset, there is now evidence to suggest that there is a profile of a survivor be it in war or catastrophe or disease. It goes without saying that physical stamina is crucial, but many times we are astonished by the fact that frail and sickly people in times of stress manage to survive while the strong and mighty quite often fall. An American psychologist, Al Siebert, participated in the Korean War and investigated the phenomenon of combat survivors.

These were soldiers who volunteered time and again for first-line combat where many or most soldiers lost their lives. These people time and again, although risking their lives, constantly managed to survive. In later years Al Siebert enlarged his work to survivors in general and not just war. After studying these people he categorised groups of assets rather than the overall profile and what comes out is that the typical survivor is a person of seemingly contradictory traits. They had a combination of being relaxed and alert, serious yet playful, focused and interested. Interested in their own survival, but also in that of others. Relaxed and alert, Siebert calls "alert-relaxation". Another word for this is playful, the ability to indulge in activity with no goal but fun or for the sole sake of curiosity. These experiences and this stored information are called upon in times of need. Actually, a survivor distinguishes himself by always being open, alert, involved and learning for the sake of learning. An ongoing process of learning and experience, all the time being at peace with himself and the world. Al Siebert reminds us, "All this cannot be taught, but it can be learnt."

*Maurice:* People often ask the question, "Does it matter in terms of my survival what my attitude is, and what my approach is at a mental level?" This is a very difficult question to answer. If you ask any doctor looking after patients with any serious illness they will mostly tell you that they intuitively feel that patients who have a positive attitude do better. At an anecdotal level we can all remember patients who seemed to be very ill and very unlikely to get through treatment and survive, who seemed to pull through on the basis of sheer willpower. There are also many situations where people who are very ill and are clearly dying manage to keep themselves going for a certain event or purpose. For example, I can remember a woman with very advanced cancer who was extremely ill and yet remained happy and symptom-free and no-one could understand how she was doing it. If you saw her walking down the street you would in no way think she was ill. Her daughter was getting married and she was looking forward to it very much. She went to the wedding, she danced, she drank, she ate, she had a thoroughly good time, she went to bed that night and died in her sleep. Under those circumstances it is difficult to get away from the feeling that she kept herself alive and feeling well through the power of her mind. Clearly that wasn't enough to make the cancer go away, but these experiences do make an impression on doctors and nurses who look after cancer patients. There is also some stronger evidence at a scientific level to support the fact that having a positive and strong fighting spirit might be important. A study was conducted in the early 1970s at Kings College

Hospital in London. In this study women who had breast cancer and had had a mastectomy as their treatment, but who had a high chance of the disease coming back, were given a questionnaire and were interviewed by a psychiatrist. They were asked a number of questions and, according to their answers, they were categorised as people who had powerful fighting spirit or who had little or no fighting spirit at all. What is very interesting is that more than 10 years later those women who had a strong fighting spirit had a greater chance of being alive and free of disease than those who were overwhelmed by the disease and who had very little fighting spirit. It was a very interesting study which is still only at the beginning of research in this area, but it suggests that fighting spirit may in some circumstances affect survival. Obviously much more work needs to be done in this area, and in fact the same group that carried out the original study is now doing further studies to look at this in a larger group of patients. Whether or not fighting spirit affects survival, there is little doubt that it improves the overall quality of life. I'll give you an example again of Vicky Clement Jones. When she was first diagnosed as having ovarian cancer in 1982 she had advanced cancer and it didn't seem likely at the time that she would live for very long. Although she initially responded well to treatment, she later on relapsed. She then carried on, despite many physical difficulties, with a very good "quality of life" for many years. She did this by always seeing the positive side of things and, as I said earlier, by always changing her expectations so that she had something to look forward to, and by setting goals which were realistic and which she could actually achieve.

**Project versus process**

*Nira:* At this point I would like to introduce you to two terms to compare and contradict them. At the end I'd like to integrate them rather than to contradict them. These terms are project versus process. A project by definition is goal-oriented behaviour where a goal decides what the best actions are to achieve that goal. On the other hand, a process is a development in which every part is a natural outcome of what went before although it may branch out and expand. So a project has a final goal right from the start, whereas a process has no final goal and the goal forms itself as it goes along. In addition a project has to focus on the goal and therefore eliminate aspects which are not directly related to that end, whereas a process simply includes what seems right while the process is taking place. The other major difference is, of course, that a project is future oriented. It aims towards achieving the goal, whereas a process concentrates on what is happening at the present time. That is to say that when we deal with a project it is important that we reach our goal and not waste time and energy on tasks which are irrelevant to the goal, not get distracted, concentrate on the end product and overcome present obstacles. During a process we might also have a general goal, but it may change as the process proceeds. So focusing on the present is more important than achieving any particular goal. I'd like to emphasise that a process does have a goal, but that the goal may well change during the process and what happens in between is more important. The major example of this of course would be life itself. If you look at life as a project then the final goal would be death and metaphorically speaking we should concentrate on death. A famous saying by a Chassidic rabbi actually says this: "One should devote all his life to prepare himself for his death." But, as we know, we use all our energy, vitality and resourcefulness not only to delay reaching that final goal, but to forget about it altogether and focus on the process which is life itself and where it is leading us.

Like life, another relevant example is cure. Now, not only life but everything in it is a process. Love is a process, cancer is a process, therapy's a process. What we are trying to introduce in this seminar are some options for improving the quality of your life and we would like you to regard the suggestions we make not as new projects to jump at, but as the beginning of a process. For every step counts, every day is a goal. What matters is how life is led rather than where it is leading to, since life is a process and needs no solutions. We are fully aware that the predominant thoughts in your mind and the ache in your stomach, the choke in the throat, means maybe one thing. Is what you're going to suggest going to cure my cancer? If so, I may just spend the rest of my life eating brown rice or doing whatever you say, but is it? In other words, is there a solution, a super solution, an ultra solution to my cancer?

What we mean by an ultra solution to cancer is a panacea, something when you take one tablet three times a day for a week and your cancer will be guaranteed to go away. There is no doubt that this is what every one of us in this room would like (though treating cancer is usually also a process). First, knowing you have cancer, your life will never be the same again. Simply from having had that knowledge, even if surgery is sufficient to completely cure the cancer and you have never had any further problems. Having faced a potentially life-threatening illness you will never see life in quite the same way again. That is not to say that this is necessarily negative, in fact, for many people they find that having been through an experience of this sort, their appreciation of life and the value and pleasure they get from what they have is much greater than it was before. For many patients with cancer, treatment involves more than a simple operation which completely removes the cancer once and for all. For many people treatment involves a series of steps, none of which can be absolutely guaranteed. Treatment therefore is more a process than a project. Ultra solutions or panaceas often don't work, although they have been the biggest ambition of human endeavour. The one ultra solution to do away with hunger, with war, with oppression and with disease is what mankind has always been searching for. When people hit a big solution, often the solution itself evokes serious problems. I try to illustrate this by a well known story from Red China. The Chinese tried an ultra solution to their demographic problem. They allowed each family to have only one child. This is very sensible, and very simple, much more effective than propaganda about birth control and family planning. This ultra solution was never tried in other cultures that face the same demographic problem.

And now years later what has happened? This ultra solution has started to backfire. They are now aware that a totally new problem is in process. Although they managed to reduce substantially the future population, this population now consists entirely of only children. Psychologically, a whole huge nation of people who think, expect, and behave like only children with all the problems that that brings. Coming back to the ultra solution, the panacea for cancer does not exist. While for some patients simple treatment is the answer, for many therapy is a process of opening new horizons. Getting there is the aim rather than being there.

## Death

*Nira:* From the moment we are aware about life, we are also aware about death. Martin Buber was quite pessimistic in many areas of life, but in this area he was very optimistic. He said that the fact that we know we are going to die in the end gives an extra meaning to our lives. If we lived for thousands of years, how would we feel about life, the image of life, the urgency of life, the need to do things in a limited time, is there an opportunity we may be missing out on? We cannot live with this awareness of death every day. We must find a balance between the fact that we know we will die one day, and yet we must live as if we will not die. Not only because we try to enjoy life, but because many of us also do things the fruit of which we will not be able to see in our lifetime.

This is part of what makes life meaningful. You do things that other people who come after you will enjoy. This gives us meaning, a way of becoming eternal.

I know that some people might be thinking, "We did not come here to discuss death. We came to this seminar to talk about how we are going to live and what we should do in order to live better and longer." There is a paradox in this. I'll give you an example. Quite a large percentage of people who commit suicide or try to commit suicide are people who are obsessed with the fear of death. They have this fear because death is the ultimate lack of control. These people feel, "I'm not going to sit in this room waiting passively for death to come and get me, the least I can do is to get out myself, I'll kill myself." It sounds paradoxical. My point is that one way of overcoming the anxiety of death is to try and experience it. We know that many people who have been near to death, whether in war, or catastrophe or car accident, often find they have overcome the anxiety of death. We can at least go through it in our mind, imagine it, live it, even for a moment, even though it may be painful to us. Now, what I would like you to do is please close your eyes. In your mind try to imagine the moment of your own death. Death can happen in many ways. It can happen to us on the road, it can happen to us in old age, surrounded by all our family. It can happen in one minute for no obvious reason, it can happen in a hospital. It can happen alone, with people, with beloved people. Some of us have always had a notion of how it is going to happen to us. Whatever comes to your mind now, whether it is an old image of yours, or you make it up now, go into the fantasy, don't be afraid of it, make friends with the fantasy. It is a fantasy. We can pick whoever we want to be with us, and however we want it to be. It's going to be our own death, the way we want it to be. Now we'll all be quiet and each of us will go into it.

**Patients and supporters commenting on their experiences**

*Trevor:* I was in our bed, in my home, with Ruth and my children and I was peaceful, not in pain, relaxed. It seems a bit naive, but that precisely was my feeling, my reaction.

*Ruth:* I'm smiling because that was exactly my situation, except that my mother came for me. I was very conscious of my mother who died 5 years ago. She was the one that appeared as though she was coming to take me somewhere, and I felt very relaxed. I had no fears and I was just very peaceful and glad that it was she who had appeared in my mind.

*Trevor:* Did it surprise you Ruth?

*Ruth:* It didn't surprise me, yet I didn't feel; I had no anger. I could see myself with Trevor and my children, who are my nearest and dearest, and yet it was strange that it was my mother that seemed to loom in front of me, and that she had come to take me with her. I don't know whether I'm surprised. It just seemed normal.

*Harry:* I was at home, in bed, it's not a new vision for me, it's part of my life, I've been there before.

About 9 months ago I was almost killed in a road accident. I was on my own in a car. In this fantasy I was killed in that accident. I have no fear of dying, only of the pain of death. I'm quite ready to go when my time comes. It was sudden, and an abrupt end to my life. I have loved fast cars and fast motor bikes for most of my life and it seemed that's the way I should have gone. But that's not the way I want to go. I was married for 28 years and my wife walked out on me, my first wife, and when she went I didn't care if I died at any time. So I went back 9 months ago, and in the fantasy I had I was killed coming home from work in that car accident. It was sudden and I was on my own.

*Beverley:* I was not in my own home, but in a country home, and I could smell the smell of the summer. It was peaceful and there were my children and Michael there and the dog, and it was just very peaceful. I could smell the country smells. I don't know if it's just because we've been walking in the country, but to me it was a relaxed and quiet time.

*Gretchen:* I could see myself from above, dying. I was in a hospital, not at home and I could see all my family there. I could see Anton and my family who are very, very close to me and it was all very peaceful. I was looking at it from above and not in the bed, looking at the people. It was a strange feeling. I felt as though I was above them watching me die, that was me in the bed, but I was above them. And it was all very peaceful.

*Gerry:* I couldn't put myself anywhere, sorry, I'll never die. I just couldn't have any vision.

*Janet:* I must be feeling the same way because I sat here and I couldn't imagine myself dying. I couldn't fantasise about myself dying. I know I'm going to die, but I've no intention of dying. I've no intention of fantasising that I am going to die. I believe that when old Gabriel blows his trumpet he'll take me away, put me in a coffin, they'll all cheer me and I'll be gone. And that'll be the end of it.

*Jane:* Well, my experience is a bit like Gretchen's. I felt as though I was viewing the whole scene from above. I was lying in my bed at home. Graham was there and our daughters, and the whole atmosphere was really quiet, relaxed and calm. You know there was no sense of fear, or panic or regret, either in them or in me. I felt that I was going into a sleep and then suddenly everything was being switched off. It just seemed a logical progression, and the people who were left didn't feel overduly sad, and it wasn't really an unpleasant picture. I always thought that if I thought of dying it would make me feel very upset, but it didn't at all.

*Tom:* I was out for a walk in the country with Margaret and the children and larking around and suddenly I died. Everything seemed to carry on. No feelings of regret or anything about it. But, nothing, no shutter came down. It just seemed to happen on a country walk, and that's it.

*Graham:* A lot of images flashed through my mind. I couldn't concentrate on a single one. I imagined being in all sorts of different environments with different situations. In some I was panicking, I found it a problem having so long to fantasise. And then I tried to imagine going through a tunnel with a light at the end, which people going through death experience and talk about. And I also tried to imagine my children as adults, but I couldn't somehow, I could imagine a sensation, but not an image.

*Vera:* Well, I was at home in bed and it was very much like going to sleep. I felt quite comfortable at the thought that I'd had enough of life and that I was ready to die. Then I imagined people around me. When it came to imagining my children, they were small and I found it really unbearable. I started visualising it all over again, with them being grown up and with me no older. That was okay, because it was like going to sleep, it was quite peaceful and all accepted.

*Rose:* I felt that I was in my own home in my own bed. It was almost as if I'd become my mother again, even though I was fairly old. Our two sons were on each side of the bed and I was trying to reassure them and say, "It's alright, it's my time to die." They were reacting with their different temperaments. Alan was weeping openly and sad, but Harry was more deeply hurt. Peter was standing behind the bed leaning over as a young man. It was peaceful. I was saying, "It's alright, it's time."

*Christopher:* I didn't experience anything much. I just had vague peaceful feelings and feelings about the countryside. That's all I remember.

*Ellen:* Well, I can't imagine myself dead, but I do know that when I die my husband will be there waiting. He had a beautiful death, he just went to sleep in my arms and all the anxiety he'd had for all those months and months disappeared. I just sat by his side, but I wasn't sad. I wasn't unhappy because he was just like he was when I met him 25 years ago. No, he just lay in my arms after he had been asleep for 5 days. He opened his eyes and looked at me like he did years and years ago, when you look at somebody with love. Everything was quiet and that anxiety was gone, he had no worries, no problems and he was at peace. That is how I hope I will die. I have this feeling that he is at peace now for the first time ever in his life, because he was always an anxious person. Knowing that he's at peace is what keeps me going. And he will be there waiting for me. I'm not waiting to go. I mean, I'm not saying, "Let it be today or tomorrow." If I'm an old lady he will be still waiting for me.

*Mave:* I imagined a big window, probably in hospital, and with my family round me, and thinking, just hoping, that you can see what's going on with your family when you've gone. Just thinking that I hope I can keep an eye on you when I'm gone. That's about it really.

*John:* It's very difficult to visualise, but I imagined that I was involved in a car crash. I was involved in one about 8 years ago which was quite minor, but I had visions of actually dying in a car crash. The ambulance came and the last thing I remember was everything going black. There was nothing else I could remember. The crash that I was involved in 8 years ago made me realise that, within split seconds, you either live or you die. That's all I can say.

*Barbara:* Mine was the same as the other two. I could see, I was looking down and seeing myself in a hospital bed surrounded by the family. I was looking down and I couldn't feel anything about being in bed. It was just peaceful with the family around.

## DAY THREE

### Family relationships – Nira with supporters

*Nira:* One group, the cancer patients, will work with Maurice, while the supporters stay in this room and work with me. But both groups will be doing the same thing. We will look at family relationships and changes in your family since you have been diagnosed as having cancer. Changes within you, within the rest of the family. We will tackle the same topics in the two groups. Let me take a couple of minutes to explain what family dynamics are. In the last few years it has become very fashionable to speak about group dynamics, family dynamics, everything has dynamics.

Let's just start to move from one person to the next. Say whatever comes to your mind. Maybe what I said triggered off something in you.

*Ellen:* I think I've been forced into a position of loyalty because my son and my husband both have cancer. My son's cancer is a malignant melanoma. He is a rather closed personality, my son, and I find it's very difficult to know what to do for him. I find I worry more about my son in a way because he's young, 36, and he's had a quite serious personality problem.

*Nira:* Can you tell us how you have been dealing with your worries?

*Ellen:* I'm not so sure that I am "dealing with them." I have this heaviness in me, an urge, a need to be doing something about my son. It has always been like that. It was never easy to talk to my son. He is a loner, but sad. I had hoped that it would change as he grew up, but it didn't. Somehow, I have this feeling that his keeping it to himself has got some relevance to his cancer. I think I should be doing something, but I don't know what to do. My loyalties are also divided. I worry more for my son, as if he is my only responsibility. That makes me feel guilty. I have always been a good wife, most of my activities were "house-wifeish". Now I have kind of lost interest in that. It didn't happen when my husband was diagnosed. It only happened when my son became sick. I have been seeing a BACUP counsellor, which has been most helpful. Even this, seeing the counsellor, like being on this weekend, is very new to me.

*Nira:* Going to see a counsellor is already a change. Losing interest in being "housewifeish" is not a loss, but rather a change of priorities. The new priorities are not yet clear, so in-between, counselling is an option. When one loses interest in one's previous way of life, there is always a worry, or even a panic, that all you will be left with is emptiness. In reality, what happened to Ellen is new, more changes will follow, and only this time in-between is empty. That's why counselling sees you through towards new directions. But not everyone switches to new goals. Some people hold on to the old plans.

*Trevor:* In our case we had quite a few things we were planning. Rather than just let it all go, we kept to our plans to sell the house, to start a new job. It's all helped to fill time and keep our minds healthy and occupied. I must say that I am not good at handling goals. When Ruth went to hospital, all I wanted was that things would stay as they were when she was home.

Ruth's a very good housekeeper, paying bills on time. I tend to open the envelope and, if it's a bill, I put it down, forget it, and then I get reminders. Ruth's much stronger on that side. When she's in hospital I feel that I should be there as much as possible, but when she comes out there's all the work and all the bills and correspondence are left. Once she's had a couple of days recuperating and starts getting a bit of her strength back it gives her something to occupy her mind. It doesn't get her down.

*Tom:* My wife has always been the major part of the family in so far as the children are concerned. But when she was in hospital I became the family, the children moved across to me. Not that they neglected their mother, but when she was well again the situation went back to what it was formerly, and when she was ill again it reversed. It's been rather confusing, this pendulum. As if the children cling to whoever is there for them.

*Nira:* In what way did it move you into the role of the father?

*Tom:* In the beginning I liked it. I always believed that it is natural for children to be attached to their mothers. When they clung to me, I was surprised. I rather expected them to wait for their mother to come back, such is their loyalty to her. In a way, it eased my worry. I cannot deny that I worry; what if, what if I will become a single parent? How would I be able to bring them up? They kind of made it simple. I don't want to indulge in this kind of thinking.

*Michael:* When my wife was in hospital there was a little vacuum which had to be filled. My children had to cling to somebody and they couldn't cling to strangers. I think there is something else which I'm sure everybody here must feel. Being overprotective, how do you stop saying "It's alright dear, I'll do it, I'll see to this, I'll see to that." My wife says, "Look, I'm not a cripple, leave me alone, let me get on with it." How do you find the fine line between caring and not being a bloody pain in the butt? You can become suffocating.

*Trevor:* I let Ruth take her normal role as soon as she feels capable of doing it. I know the sort of person she is when she is fit enough to do it, she's got to do it. She'll do it and I'll just let her get on with it. I'd help her but I let her do what she thinks she can do. I won't be overprotective.

*Anton:* I share the beliefs of Michael about the vacuum. I fell into the vacuum and I thoroughly enjoyed it. I wish I could take on the role. In November and December of last year when Gretchen was in hospital, I just gave up everything and just concentrated on the home; everything was great. I felt in total control. Now it is different, she's come out and she fills in that vacuum. I moved back and made some money. I feel as though she and I are fighting cancer together and I sometimes wish I could share the pain with her. I could have it 6 months and she could have it 6 months.

My anxieties at the moment are practical ones, but I believe there's more underneath that. I know that I can give enough love to the children.

We both have always given them love and they respect and love us equally. I know I can do that, but I can't do that and earn x thousands pounds a year. So I know I'm going to have to delegate. I know I'm going to have to have au pairs, minders, chauffeurs; they're the practical and physical anxieties, which I think I can overcome. And I'm going to overcome them with money.

*Tom:* I can understand what he's saying to a degree. In my case, when Margaret got the disease, I did have anxiety. I admit that I've still got it now. I've got that anxiety inside, exactly as you were saying. I am anxious that at some stage I will have to carry out the role that Margaret's been carrying out so far.

*Trevor:* As far as I'm concerned, I'm a provider, and because I'm a provider people expect me to carry on in the normal way I've been carrying on and provide for my family unit. Now that to me has been a very, very difficult thing to do because there aren't enough hours in the day. I've had to look after the family, I've had to go to work and try to do my work in the normal way. People have helped me at work, but they still expect me to do my day's jobs and then, at the end of that day, rush off to the hospital because I want to see my wife and make sure everything's well. Then I go home and see to the children. Then I start again the next day, and that's an anxiety in itself, the fact that I've got to keep going.

*Graham:* I am an optician, so I have treated people for many years. When Jane was hospitalised, I experienced, after a while, a kind of depression unfamiliar to me. Only much later I understood how all these things affected me. It all started with the daily visits to the hospital. First of all you have all experienced that hour in a hospital which seems to last a lot longer. It is terribly tiring to sit in a hospital. You forget about time, it seems to last forever. Even though you have spent an hour with the person you came to visit they would say it had been a very short while. The day in the hospital is very long. One hour is a very tiny part of this 24-hour day in hospital. For you to spend an hour in a hospital often means 3 hours, including travelling time, so a 1-hour visit may be 3 hours out of your day. You know that you're already late for your children who have been neglected, so you feel guilty again and you feel you are in a losing situation. You are not going well in your job, you don't spend enough time in the hospital, you do the shopping on the way home, the children are crying and are hungry and you never get time to yourself. What about you and the fatigue that is accumulating?

*Nira:* We can carry on in automatic pilot for a long time. So what do you do? The one thing you can allow yourself is to break down physically. Morally you are not supposed to collapse. So the next thing that happens is fatigue, depression, incompetence. You start to forget things. You become a little indifferent. This is why you should avoid getting to this point. Some people, when they get to this point, take a very long time to get out of it. They become the patient. After a short while you have to organise your life and give yourself a proper respectful place within that new organisation. You cannot put the patient in the centre, because paradoxically for them it is often becoming easier. The children are taken care of, so are the house chores. Paradoxically, it's easier, but you are now in severe stress. You are not competent enough to carry out your additional roles because you are always late for what you are doing and you are not doing it well enough. You have to respect yourself. Some people find it very difficult to say to a cancer patient, "I'm very tired, I don't think I'll come to the hospital tomorrow. Tomorrow I'm taking off. I think I'll sleep in the afternoon."

*Vera:* I think you're absolutely wrong. It's impossible. I would feel very guilty because I was putting myself above somebody who was really sick. I couldn't put myself in the role where my wellbeing was more important. I don't think any of us could. I think that's theorising.

*Michael:* It may have to do with a particular person's metabolism. You keep going because you keep going. The drive and the tension and the additional nervous energy keep you going. I think if I slackened and I stopped, I would probably crumble.

*Nira:* But you don't have to stop. Just rest and energise. Even you cannot go on forever. With cancer you never know how long a person may be ill. Some people put in a big effort over a short time and then collapse. Other people can carry on, and on, because they also know how to relax, how to rest, how to become equal and say, "Today I'm not coming to the hospital."

Some of you have the idea that it's a competitive situation. It's either you or her. It seems like an either/or situation, but it's not like that, and it should not be like that. We are trying not to come to the point where one person has to be selfless, or make sacrifices if you want an even more dramatic word. Why? Because it doesn't work. Resentment and anger accumulate and the other person will sense it because resentment is not something that we can hide. The whole idea of the dynamics of a personality is that whatever you have inside shows. You cannot hide it. That's why I said, don't make yourself a victim. Victimisation doesn't pay, doesn't work, and that's why you have to respect yourself too.

*Tom:* One of the resentments that I have, which has come out of this situation, is the fact that now Margaret considers that because she's got this cancer, everything else is insignificant. I've had the flu recently and, to her, this is minimal because she's got a disease which is an ongoing thing. Anything less than that is nothing at all and she passes it off quite dismissively.

*Michael:* Recently when I had flu I was off for three weeks and I actually passed out at one stage. My wife picked me up and looked after me and everything. Once someone has cancer everything else in the normal run of the mill seems to be minimal. I also get the feeling that I can't share with her until it actually happens to me. I try hard to understand and to be supportive and I try to be as natural as possible, but there are times when we both grate against each other because she's in a different situation to me.

*Graham:* I'll go back 6 years ago. I had a good job in industry and jacked it in and went off to University in Manchester to do a degree in optics and now I'm an optician. So that threw on Jane the role of being the breadwinner of the family and, in a way, the leader, while I was away. I went off to Manchester during the week and came home at weekends. Jane chose to get her own private physiotherapy business going and also to do an Open University degree which put terrific stress on her, so what I did may have caused the stress which resulted in the cancer that she had. Now I'm established as a qualified optician, I want to start up my own practice; it could be anywhere in the country, but if I uproot her, am I going to cause stress again and cause the cancer to come back? I feel guilty thinking about it. We need to communicate and Jane's not a good communicator. She bottles things up, she's very bright and cheerful on the surface, but bottles things up underneath. I'm in the situation where I feel I caused her terrific stress which could have resulted in the cancer.

*Ellen:* I didn't know how to bring this up in the group, since I have never really fully admitted it to myself. I, too, like Graham, feel that in a way I have given Chris his cancer. In the early years he used to get really angry at my incompetence. When he insulted me, I was cross with him for days and days. I rejected him, and he felt lonely. I, too, felt lonely, but I couldn't tolerate his language. I come from a family where people respect each other. He made me feel very upset with myself. True, he is very hard working and competent, and many people cling to him, out of a need for him. While I just do my secretarial job. It seems unfair that it happened to him. He is needed much more than I am. I feel guilty because of the early years, I also think, "I should be the one, why him?" I hate this kind of thinking, I know it is wrong, if I go on it may make me sick as well.

*Peter:* I don't believe that anyone can give you cancer. This just happens. I also felt it unfair to Rose. Why her? But when I think about the future, it's then that I feel kind of guilty, but mostly I feel pain. I know that the business we have both worked on will be OK in the future. Also I believe that our sons, who are now at university, will be fine, and Rose won't be there with me to enjoy all that. Rose has advanced cancer, and even now, when she was back from the hospital, she came in to give a hand with the business.

*Ellen:* Chris is also very ill. We are both fighting it as best we can, but I am becoming more and more anxious, I am not myself. In spite of my anxiety, I find it hard, even now, to ignore Chris's behaviour at home. He is taking even more liberties now, and is leaving things all over the place, as if nothing matters at all. I know that it should not bother me, like when I come home from work at 6 o'clock, and he has been all day at home, and the sink is filled with dishes. I can hardly hold my anger.

*Graham:* I have tried hard to take every day as it comes. I know that this is what we should be doing, but it doesn't work. Since the first time that the doctor said, "It's cancer", I have been obsessed with my fear of Jane's dying, and of my being alone for the rest of my life. I know I would never want another woman. Jane and I go back a long way, she is my best friend: my only friend. I tried to use my imagination, but I was never very good at it. All I see for myself is darkness. I've never been alone. My only hope is that, in the end, Jane will not leave me alone. She cannot .... It may sound strange to you, but this has been inside me for a long time. This is the first time that I have spoken about it.

*Nira:* Guilt is inherent in human nature, and this is part of what makes us human. We have shared here different expressions of guilt that have in common what is known as "survivor's guilt". Part of the meaning of life is a belief in some plan, a superior order, that punishes and rewards us for our behaviour. We all say, "such is life", meaning that things happen. But, in our heart of hearts, we pray to be spared. We deserve it because we have been good, hard working, kindly people, etc., etc. Only when it happens to our loved ones do we realise that our secret prayers have been answered and we were spared, and we feel guilty that perhaps we have somehow arranged it. Soldiers who survive battles where most people have been killed suffer from this guilt. Holocaust survivors suffer from it, and families of cancer patients, as well as many others, also suffer from it.

Being a supporter for many is a whole new experience. The less you feel guilty, the more normally you behave, the better it is for the family.

Not being angry over the full sink is abnormal. The familiar anger over mundane matters is reassuring that life is going on the way it should be. Can turning the situation into a privilege, as one of you so directly said yesterday, mean "You are your brother's keeper?"

## Maurice with patients

*Maurice:* Have your relationships changed since having cancer?

*Beverley:* I think what happened in my relationship with Michael is that although we have always enjoyed a very good marriage, cancer has brought us closer together because of all the problems that came with it. Our children are grown up and don't live with us, so our immediate support is from each other. Although we have, thank God, two wonderfully supportive children; my son, who's 27, likes to talk about everything connected with my problem, whereas my daughter who is 25, and married, prefers not to talk about it; she'll accept but she doesn't really want to know. That's her way of coping. Everybody copes in a different way. Michael is very strong.

My interests have changed and that has affected some aspects of our relationship. Michael talks about something that's going to happen in 10 years' time and I switch off at that because I think to myself, well that's a load of rubbish, how do I know I'm going to be here in 10 years' time? I'm only interested in the immediate, in within a short space of time. I plan positively for 6 months or a year, and take that in my stride. I'm not interested in planning for things years hence when he's going to be retired and so forth, because that to me is totally unimportant. It's the now that's important, everything that happens, and the pleasures that are available and to be enjoyed at the moment.

Before I had cancer, one used to think, in the normal married way, of when we were going to be possibly in a financial situation to do x, y, z, when you're going to travel more and when you're going to retire. For example, we thought of living abroad. That is a certain change in my life now because I'm not interested. I'm only interested in now.

*Jane:* I think probably before I had cancer I was the one who was perhaps the more nurturing one. I was always very cheery and bright and Graham used to get depressed at times; he's that sort of person. I was always the one who was jollying things along. I think that has really changed now; since I had cancer he is always so positive and cheerful, and supports me much more in that way. I suppose it was a strange situation because he was at university for 4 years doing a second degree just before I got cancer, and I was doing all the breadwinning, and taking all the responsibilities. He was very involved in his course and wasn't really interested. I suppose at that time I was forced into a much more dominant role in the home which I didn't really like very much. Now I've sort of dropped that. Fortunately he finished his degree course just about the time I was diagnosed so that was lucky. Now he has taken many more of the responsibilities and I feel much better. He has been very supportive and encouraged me to do all those things that I want to do, and I think the main thing is, we are much closer. We always had a happy marriage, but we are much more demonstrative towards each other now. We hug each other a lot more and we talk a lot more about things. We communicate a great deal more than we used to. I used to think our marriage was happy, but looking back over the last year, it's so much better now. We're much more on the same wavelength and much, much closer emotionally. I think that's the main change, really.

*Margaret:* I'm the opposite, I don't feel we communicate enough. I think I take an awful lot on myself. I think I was on my own for years with my three children. We were all very close; even though they've grown up they are very dependent on me for anything in their life. They're on the 'phone or they come round and they want me and I've always been there. I find now that I've got cancer we don't communicate very well. He'll take me everywhere, on holiday, yes, fill our lives with everything that we can possibly do. We've been away and, if I wanted to go away next weekend, fine, we'd go, but I don't feel that is enough for me. Since I have had cancer I can talk more to our children. They're around every day and every evening saying "How are you?" and I can discuss anything with them, but I find I don't discuss it with Tom as much.

I feel he is trying to fill my life with all the things that he feels money can buy. I didn't feel he was able to talk to me to make me feel better. I didn't get any joy out of him coming in and talking to me, it didn't make me feel good, whereas my children could come in and I would feel better. In the past we would talk about what we were going to do in the future. I suddenly lost that with him. We were going to retire and go to the country and all that. I don't talk about this any more, so suddenly we've lost all the things that we had planned for the future. Suddenly I find that we'll spend hours without talking; there's probably an awful lot going round in my mind, and I don't bother to talk about it any more. I wouldn't say he doesn't understand about cancer, but perhaps it's something inwardly that I'm keeping to myself. Because I haven't got somebody I can express it to. So it has definitely changed. We would talk for hours before.

*Maurice:* What would you like him to say to you when you talk about how you're feeling about the cancer? What would you like that you're not getting?

*Margaret:* I think I'd like him to make me feel that there is a future, that I am going to be cured.

*Maurice:* What are the words that your children use that he doesn't use? What makes the difference?

*Margaret:* I think they're much more bubbly and much more down to earth, whereas Tom is very, very quiet. He really thinks about his words; he doesn't walk in and say, "Hallo, how are you, you look great", he hasn't got that manner. He wasn't like that ever before.

*Maurice:* You didn't need it before.

*Margaret:* No, I didn't need it, that's right. My relationship with my children has improved a lot. Before I was always the one who was supportive, now they're the other way. They support me. They really are wonderful. If there's a hospital appointment they take a day off from work. They're with me much more than Tom.

*Maurice:* Do you respond differently to different children?

*Margaret:* Oh yes, yes. I've got a younger one that takes an awful lot in but she doesn't say anything. She is really quiet and doesn't express her feelings.

*Maurice:* And how does she affect you?

*Margaret:* I feel sometimes she doesn't care at all because she is so quiet. I think, "Well, why the hell don't you sort of feel something?" She doesn't bother to put herself out to do anything, but the other two are so different.

*Maurice:* In what way are they different?

*Margaret:* Well, they would come in and say, "Do you want a cup of tea?" and put the kettle on. They would do something. I don't want sympathy, don't get me wrong, I don't need that, but it's nice to think they're there to help. Now, instead of me doing everything for them, it's great that they have turned the other way round. The younger one doesn't really do anything. She doesn't say anything either.

*Maurice:* Would it be true that there are some similarities to the way she relates to you, and the way that Tom relates to you?

*Margaret:* That's right.

*Maurice:* And you have difficulty with the situation where somebody is not expressing what they're thinking. What you just said is that if she doesn't talk to you, there is a feeling from your point of view that she isn't bothering.

*Margaret:* That she doesn't care, yes.

*Maurice:* Perhaps you feel something similar with Tom.

*Margaret:* I know Tom does care.

*Maurice:* So what you're saying is that if somebody doesn't express things to you in a verbal and direct way, then you look at them and you read their minds, and automatically the thought that comes to your mind is that they don't care.

*Margaret:* That's right, and it doesn't bring the best out in me because it makes me close in.

*Maurice:* Yes, and so you react in a way that says, "He doesn't care about me", or your daughter doesn't care about you, yet you know they do care. But something about the way they relate to you makes you feel that.

*Jane:* My experience has been quite similar. I feel that we have been drawn apart the whole time since I have been diagnosed with cancer. I feel it hasn't been a shared experience between us. Graham's reaction to my having cancer was that I was going to get well and he wasn't going to worry. My reaction was that I would die from having cancer the way my mother died. However much I tried to contort myself into feeling positive and optimistic about it, I just didn't. I needed to make space for my feelings of depression and desperation. I still feel that is probably a more realistic reaction to having cancer. The people whom I stayed close to during the last few months were friends who actually faced up to their own anxieties about cancer and who would talk to me about death and dying, and not people who would say, "You've got to fight it", and all that. That was my initial reaction, but I just didn't find it appropriate after a while. I did feel it would offer me some degree of control over the cancer which made it quite attractive. Then I found it all getting very oppressive and it didn't feel right for me.

*Maurice:* So you felt that your relationship with Graham became more distant because he was saying, "Be positive and you'll be alright", while you wanted to feel that he understood more about what you were going through, that he could share your anxiety, rather than just encourage you?

*Jane:* I mean our relationship wasn't very good before my having cancer, but it became more distant after I got cancer.

*Beverley:* All of my family have been supportive. My brother and sister-in-law nursed their son through 2 years of leukaemia and then he died the week before I was diagnosed. They were helpful to me because I could talk to them, and my sister-in-law knew a lot of things having been in Addenbrookes for 2 years, so they were very supportive. The relationship with my husband is closer together. We had a good marriage beforehand, and we're even closer now. He's had to take on a lot more. I previously always saw to things in the house.

*Christopher:* My situation is a little bit different from everybody else around here because my family is grown up. I was married at an early age and have two children, our son is 36, and our daughter 27. I started in 1980 with cancer and fortunately I've never been hospitalised. It's always been going to Doncaster Royal Infirmary on a day basis, taking drugs and going through it that way. I've always been the breadwinner, and that is always at the back of my mind, what happens if I get to a position where I can't work? My wife had to finish work in 1979 through her health problems.

*Beverley:* Michael is the most supportive person I could ever want around me. He's generally the only person I prefer to have around me and our relationship has just got closer since the whole cancer business started. He's been the ultimate support, and everything I could ever want.

There was a time when I first had cancer that he wanted to close up all the family, close the door and not let anybody in, just say, "Right, I'm going to sort this lot out myself. I'll look after the family, I'll look after the kids and I'll look after Beverley." I thought, well what's going on? We need everybody we can lay our hands on. All of a sudden he was trying to sweep everybody away, but I think he did get over that and realised that it was impossible for him, and allowed the family back in. Our relationship hasn't suffered at all, it's brought us closer together.

*Mave:* When I was diagnosed my husband and I had been together 10 or 12 years. There had been other things in our lives together which have been catastrophes, and this seemed to be just another one. We've got a strategy for dealing with crises. This was another crisis which we would face together. I don't think there have been any essential changes in our relationship, but there have been big changes in my relationship with the rest of the world. That was the biggest change, because to the rest of the world, before this happened, I'd been the confident one, the one that everybody turned to when they had problems, and I had to learn to be the weak one. My initial reaction when I was diagnosed was that I didn't want to see anybody; didn't want to deal with anybody because I could only deal with them in a supportive role. In the first few days everybody was so shocked and so upset that I had to support them. I also had to learn to be weak, to say to people, "I'm bewildered, I'm upset by this", and that was something I'd never done before. It has been a valuable lesson because a lot of people have become a lot closer to me because of it.

*John:* Some friends can't cope and their reaction is, "You're going to get better", and they emphasise the positive side. You just cannot talk to them. That's their coping strategy. Some of these people are quite close to me. That's what they want and that is fine, but we're not communicating, so the relationship is in some ways dead. The people to whom I can confide things that I've never confessed before, like my weaknesses, have been very valuable. They in turn confess their weaknesses to me and we're just closer.

*Mave:* Certainly the biggest change for me was to learn how to be weak to the rest of the world.

## Children

*Graham:* Can I ask just for a general bit of advice, I think for other people in the room as well? About children; this is a concern for Jane and me. We have two children, aged 8 and 4. I like to think that we know how to communicate with them, and we know what to say to them and when. We seem to be doing a fairly good job, but would like advice from you, Nira.

*Nira:* I would like to comment on that. The best example is sex; when we want to explain to young children about sex, many parents are very embarrassed about how to go about it. There's no need. Children who ask about sex are very satisfied when you give them the exact answer to the question they asked. This is a step-by-step process. Children don't see the big picture, so you answer each question one at a time.

*Christopher:* We made a policy years ago never to mention cancer, so we mention "disease, illness, or sickness". We don't use the word cancer because of the bad PR it's got. Kids can pick up gossip.

*Ruth:* My little girl actually came up to me when she saw me with no hair and she said "This cancer's very bad isn't it?" She just accepts it. She writes about it in her school work and she tells her friends. Because other children say "Your Mum's always wearing a hat", she just tells them.

*Janet:* I would worry about that. I don't want that because I feel it would be a burden on the child. You know that it wouldn't take too long for the child to get to know that cancer may mean, possibly, death. I wouldn't want my child to go around with that sort of burden.

*Margaret:* Well our children have seen their cousin die. They wanted to know everything. They weren't allowed to go to his funeral; that weighed on our son's mind, so we took him to the cemetery. He was expecting to see him, so now everything is open.

*Gretchen:* I believe that cancer is only a word, it's nothing else. The disease will still be there whatever you want to call it. We feel that our children should know about it as and when they ask and we shouldn't suppress that word because it is still called cancer.

*Nira:* I want to make another point. If you have cancer, something has happened to you that changed your life. It also changed the life of your husband or wife. It also changed the life of your children, even if they are only 4 years old, you cannot deny that. So they should know what it is and not be afraid of it. It happened to them too. Just like divorce. It is better to give them an explanation about what is happening to them because children of divorced parents have to face the world. You know, 20 years ago divorce was bad PR too. Today, it is common, but you become a certain kind of person when you are a child of divorced parents. You have to defend yourself against these attitudes, so the better ammunition you have for this defence the better you are equipped. Information is important, but how much information depends on the child. When mum and dad are having a row there is one child that goes under the blanket and covers himself, he doesn't want to listen, it is too alarming. Another child will come round and try to be the mediator, so they have different personalities. That goes for cancer, too. One child doesn't want to know, another wants to know everything. Maurice, I know you want to come in on that.

*Maurice:* I've a friend from California, where in Los Angeles the divorce rate is extremely high. Many people get divorced several times. He has not been divorced and he was telling me that his children at school are the odd ones out by far. It was a sort of status symbol amongst the children to brag about how many times their parents had been divorced. And the children actually felt to some extent left out that their parents had never been divorced even once. The other thing I just wanted to comment about – I have a daughter, Lindi, who is 12, and another, Amy, who is 9 – when the older one was 8 there was a programme at school where children were warned not to go off with strangers. They also took it one step further and said the children should create a secret password. This password would be something that only they and their mother and father would know, so if some day your mum couldn't come and get you because she was delayed and she had to send a stranger, the stranger would use the password. It sounded like a very sensible idea, so my daughter Lindi came to me and she said, "I've got a great password that I told my teacher today." The word she chose was "cancer". I didn't talk to my daughter of 8 about cancer, but she clearly has a different view growing up with a cancer doctor. I talk to a lot of people about what to tell their children about cancer and I get a lot of feedback. I'm always interested to know what happened when they told their children. There are two main areas of difficulty.

The first is explaining to children about cancer. In my experience how children take it depends on how you explain it to them. I'm sure if you explain it with tremendous anxiety they will pick up that anxiety, but if you explain it to them in a simple and relaxed way, they take it in the same way. What you tell them depends on the age of the child. Even young children will understand that the body's made of tiny little things called cells, that they are like bricks that make a wall, but they're very, very small and you can't see them. You can talk to young children about good cells and bad cells and explain that bad cells form lumps, and as a result of those lumps they make mummy sick. They will understand that she is having treatment to make the lumps go away, that the treatment makes her sick, that the reason her hair has fallen out is because of the treatment and that it will grow back again. Older children and teenagers understand quite complex information. The feedback I get from people is that they're always stunned by how little their children are disturbed or upset by this information.

The other problem area is talking to children about death. How do you convey this to a child? Some people feel it's a very bad thing to discuss with a child that their parent might be dying. The problem is that if someone does die, there is no doubt the children are eventually going to be aware of it. My experience is that it is best to tell children in stages. If somebody's going into hospital very often you can explain that mummy's getting sicker and has to spend more time in hospital. You can later go on to explain that mummy cannot come home and, still later, talk about her dying. It is a great help not only to tell them that she's dying, but to give them an opportunity to discuss it with their mother. You can actually talk about where you go when you die and what you say depends on your beliefs. Children often ask the questions directly. A number of studies show that many children blame themselves for their parent's cancer or even their parent's death. It may be important to reassure the child it has nothing to do with them. Entering into a dialogue with children is very, very helpful. There are also some lovely little books which are available, which actually talk about dying in terms children can understand. One is *Badger's Parting Gift* (Varley 1985), and the others are *Grandpa and Me* (Alex and Alex 1981) and *Charlotte's Web* (White 1969), three stories which put death in a beautiful way specifically for children. These books can act as a very useful starting point for a discussion.

*Beverley:* I agree with you that everybody's got their own way of communicating with their children, whether it's about sex or anything else. We've all got our own techniques and we think we're good at them, but our fear is that if we go all the way with them it will be a playground conversation. It will be, "My grandma died of cancer yesterday", and I can just see Nicky asking the ultimate question, "Cancer kills, doesn't it? Does that mean mummy's going to die?" So I'm immediately then faced with the ultimate question.

*Nira:* I would like to come in here. You'd be surprised what your children know at that stage. Even without you telling them. Because children pick up things and are very sensitive. You can see that in their drawings and in their stories, what they know of what's going on in the family, including disease. That's why it is important to speak to them. Because anxiety is much worse than accurate knowledge. What they pick up makes them more anxious than if you gave them the information yourself.

*Maurice:* I think we all underestimate just how strong our children are, and how much they already know. And they usually already do know. Children are helped a lot by knowing in advance what might happen. If they ask whether Mummy might die of the cancer you can say "A person can die of cancer, but we hope things will be fine." At a later stage you might say "It is possible mummy might die." Put them on the bed and talk about it, and discuss their fears of death. Not only is it good for the children, but it's good for you.

*Beverley:* I think you're wrong that we underestimate our children. We're realistic, everyone should be realistic about it. And in communicating with the children I've always felt it's important that the quality of the information is at a level that they can, in fact, understand. So one would, in fact, use language that related to the language they use and the experiences they've had. I think also that the other important thing is the attitude that we have, that we're courageous in our attitude and positive and hopeful about what is going to happen. The child will pick that up.

*Nira:* Part of what children suffer is called "survivors' guilt". You know children have dreams about their parents. They have anger and sometimes might wish mummy dead, and then when she becomes ill or dies the feeling is, "I caused it." Young children have what is called magical thinking. That I have powers, I can do it. If you don't see me, I don't see you; magical thinking. What you imagine eventually happens and they feel they caused it. So children have fears of losing their parents which have nothing to do with cancer. What do I do if you die?

And we answer that straight. At a certain age, say 4 years old, children ask very often, "Mummy, do you love me?" There is only one good answer to this question, "No." Their response is, "Mummy, I don't believe you", and then you say, "Silly questions get silly answers." You can answer many times, "I love you, I love you dearly", and they then repeat, "Mummy, do you love me?" This is a little power game. The child knows that you are vulnerable when they ask this question. Of course they know you love them. They respond to a challenge.

I suggest you go about it this way, "If I die it is very sad, but there are solutions and you will be alright."

*Janet:* It seems to me there are lots of very good reasons why a child should feel guilty. If someone's ill in bed and you naturally tell a child not to disturb them, you know they will still be noisy and so on, so when something does happen, it's not surprising that they then feel a sense of guilt. That leads me to another question. You said it is sufficient to answer their questions, but how do you know that they will ask the questions? Don't you think they might build up an anxiety, so they don't actually ask you what is on their mind?

*Nira:* That's part of your relationship with your child. I mean, do you communicate? That's communication. And you sense what a child has in mind and then you give the child an opening and sometimes he picks it up, sometimes he doesn't. Sometimes you volunteer information even if it is not asked, because you see it is on his mind.

*Maurice:* You often pick up what is happening with children, not by what they say but by the way they are behaving. You notice they are "naughty" or irritable, or uncooperative, or they regress, e.g. to bed wetting.

*Gretchen:* I've stood at the back of a crowded bus and sudden deathly silence descended when my 6-year-old asked, "Why did you get cancer mum?" That was a natural question to her. She was at the age when it was a string of questions, one after the other. The rest of the bus froze, but to her it was a natural question.

## What you can do to help yourself

*Maurice:* There are a number of things at a practical level that experience over the years has shown people with cancer and their relatives that they can do to help themselves. What do I mean by helping yourself? Obviously for everybody here the help that you want is advice on how to overcome your cancer. If you go to one of the alternative therapists, they may be able to tell you confidently that if you do this or that and behave in a particular way, or follow a certain diet or resolve your emotional difficulties, your cancer will go away. Nira and I come from the conventional school and we have no intention of making exaggerated claims which cannot be substantiated. The things we are going to suggest are those things which you can do which will improve your general overall state of health and quality of life both physically and emotionally. We know from experience that people who decide to do something for themselves usually develop a more positive attitude, feeling that they have regained control over their lives, and we discussed the importance of that earlier. In Britain many doctors intuitively believe that patients with a strong fighting spirit may also have a better outlook. This is very difficult to prove, although I have mentioned some research from Kings College Hospital and the Royal Marsden Hospital which has suggested that positive fighting spirit could possibly affect survival. Getting yourself as physically and mentally fit as possible can only be helpful in fighting any illness. Nira has also discussed the philosophy of the "wisdom of the desert", that resolving problems rarely takes place at the level of the problem and sometimes the most effective way of solving an issue which you are finding difficult is to do it indirectly.

There are five areas we are going to discuss where you may be able to do things to help yourself. It may well be that you can find other areas which would be particularly helpful to you.

The first area I want to discuss is that of diet. There is now quite a lot of evidence to suggest that diet may play a role in causing cancer. Sir Richard Doll, epidemiologist, has suggested that somewhere between 30 and 50 per cent of cancer may be caused by diet. That is to say that our diet over our whole lives may affect our risk of cancer. Now how do scientists come to this conclusion? Obviously you can't divide the population into two halves, give one half of them a particular diet over 30 years and the other half a different diet and then see what happens with the amount of cancer they get. The only way you can do it is to look at whole populations and see what cancers they get, have a look at their diet and see if there are other factors which could also influence this. An example of this sort of study is if you look at Japan and you will find that there is a very high risk of stomach cancer, but a low risk of breast cancer compared, for example, to the United States, where breast cancer is the commonest cancer in women and stomach cancer is much less common. There are obviously two possibilities for this; it could be a genetic difference or it could be an environmental one. It is, of course, very interesting to look at the Japanese who emigrated to the United

States, who didn't marry Americans but married other Japanese. If you look at their children and grandchildren you find that the risk of stomach cancer has decreased to be much more like that of the Americans, while the risk of breast cancer has increased. It is thought that these differences can probably be explained by differences in diet. Another example is in Central Africa where the diet is very high in fibre and low in fat and what you find is that colon cancer is virtually unknown and breast cancer is uncommon. And if you look at populations where the diet is high in fat and low in fibre, the risk of these cancers is much greater.

The basic principles for a healthy diet which might decrease our risk of a cancer are the same principles which would reduce the risk of heart disease and diabetes, so eating a good healthy diet can only be helpful.

Although what I've just said strongly suggests that if the population were to eat a different diet the amount of cancer they get would probably be lower, that is not the same as saying that if you change your diet once you've got cancer that will make it go away. This is the major point of difference with some of the alternative therapies and the attitude of the conventional physician. If you go to an alternative cancer centre many of the dietary suggestions they make would not be very different from the ones that I am going to suggest other than being more radical. The major difference would be in the promises they made. They may tell you with confidence that if you followed this principle your cancer would go away. Unfortunately, cancer doesn't work like that. If that were the case, lung cancer would go away if people stopped smoking once they had found out the diagnosis, and clearly it doesn't. But eating a good generally healthy diet can only improve your general state of health and be helpful in fighting any illness.

So what are the principles of a healthy diet? They are, in fact, very simple. The first is to eat more fresh fruit, fresh vegetables and cereals and grains. That does two things. First it gives you the right sort of carbohydrates, the type that you find in fruit and vegetables rather than the unhealthy sort of carbohydrates found predominantly in sweets and cakes. In addition to that, they contain a lot of fibre which is an important component of a healthy diet. The emphasis is on changing slowly, perhaps considering having breakfast cereal such as muesli, eating some fresh fruit and making sure you have vegetables every day. In addition to this you reduce the amount of sweets and cakes that you eat. Once again, the emphasis is on doing this slowly.

The second is to eat less red meat and to have more chicken and fish instead. This doesn't mean that you go to extremes and stop eating all red meat and eat only chicken or fish; eat slightly less red meat and more chicken and fish. It is important to do things slowly and not to make radical or dramatic changes immediately. Many people who try to make these changes give up after the first few days. On the other hand, if they do things slowly, slowly incorporating them into their lives, the changes are more likely to be permanent.

These are the major principles of a healthy diet. Of course, if you are significantly overweight it is sensible to try and reduce your weight to a reasonable level.

The next thing I want to talk about that can help you improve the way you relate to yourself and your own self-image, as well as how you feel physically and mentally, is the question of exercise. Exercise is something which we can all do to help ourselves improve the quality of our lives. What I mean by exercise is anything which suits you and which can be done on a regular basis. I don't think it's a good idea to suddenly get up tomorrow morning at 5a.m. and run 5 miles. What is important is to do something on a regular basis which you start off slowly and build up slowly. With exercise if you do too much too quickly you can deplete your energy rather than increase it. As with every one of these things we don't want you to make any dramatic changes, but to build in changes which take place at a slow pace. So what you can do will depend on how physically fit you are at the moment. You might decide that you are going to start off by walking 100 yards three times a week. Other people might feel they can walk a mile at a brisk pace and that would be a reasonable place for them to start. The best thing to do is allocate a period of time, say 20 minutes three times a week, where you decide that you will actually try to do some exercise. Now at the beginning, if you are physically unfit, that 20 minutes might be 5 minutes walking, 5 minutes resting and 5 minutes walking and 5 minutes resting. As you slowly get fitter you will find that the period of the exercise will become longer and periods of rest shorter. For some people exercise might be going to a gym, for others it might be swimming, walking or running; for others it might be strolling in the park. With any regular exercise you will find that you slowly increase the amount of energy you have, you will improve what you look like, you'll be more trim, more fit, and will enjoy life more. You obviously need to discuss what exercise you do with your doctor. In general, it is unlikely to be harmful. The main principle to bear in mind when starting off is exercise within the limits of what you can do comfortably without exhausting yourself. In general, you are unlikely to harm yourself doing that, but you should just discuss it with your doctor before you start.

I am now going to get on to the question of relaxation. Once again the same principle applies. You want to start off slowly with the aim of trying to incorporate some form of relaxation on a regular basis into your life. This is not something which will suit everybody. For some people they will find that half an hour every day in the bath filled with bath salts, just allowing yourself to soak and to forget about what's going on in your life, is excellent relaxation. For others, listening to music on a regular basis clears your mind of all other thoughts and provides all the relaxation that you need. The picture of the man coming home from work every day, sitting down in front of the fire, having his slippers and a large cigar brought to him is relaxing just to think about. I had a patient who tells me that when he takes the first puff of a cigar at the end of the day he immediately relaxes. As a cancer doctor I am not going to suggest you smoke a cigar every day, but I would guess that one cigar a day probably does you a lot less harm than not having that period of relaxation. Other people find weeding the garden, playing with their children, doing crossword puzzles, relaxes them. Another way of achieving the feeling of relaxation on a regular basis is to do relaxation exercises. There are a number of tapes available and even classes that you can attend which will teach you to do this and carrying out these relaxation exercises several times a week can bring a degree of peace into your life. There are a number of studies which show that regular relaxation not only reduces anxiety and depression, but can also control symptoms such as pain, nausea and vomiting.

Many people ask about meditation, yoga and so on. These techniques are merely other ways of achieving a peaceful, relaxed state of mind. We often speak about music being what we call meditative. I think for many people the term "meditation" invokes connotations of an Eastern philosophy which is difficult for them to get into, but if that is something which suits you and which you feel comfortable with, then any of these techniques can be helpful to achieve a relaxed, peaceful state of mind which will contribute to your quality of life.

The next topic I would like to discuss is that of play and fun. Now we often think of playfulness and fun as something for children and not something for serious adults. Yet if we think back to the last time we got involved in a lighthearted playful situation which had no purpose other than just the fun of messing around, you will remember how energetic and cheerful you felt afterwards. The problem for many of us is that we are so serious about getting on with our work, achieving what we strive for, be it progress in our career, getting a new house, making money or overcoming a cancer, that we forget how important and essential it is to have play in our lives. Play is simply something which is conducted for the activity itself without any purpose, without there being any outcome. So, if you decide that you like juggling with two balls, this will be relaxing and fun till such time as you become ambitious and set yourself targets and continually try to improve the standard or your juggling.

What about the people in your lives? I am sure we have all had the experience of walking down the street and seeing someone at 200 yards and immediately feeling happy at seeing them. You stop and chat for a few minutes about virtually nothing and you walk off feeling better because you have spoken to him. Another time you see someone at 200 yards and you immediately feel "Oh God", and your heart sinks. You have a brief chat, and nothing much is said, but you somehow feel uneasy and ill at ease. They ask you how you are and, for no good reason, you feel inadequate and awkward. There is nothing sinister about the second person, they just have that effect on you.

Most people in our lives can simply be divided into those with whom we feel good, people who nurture us, and those who make us feel bad about ourselves, people who have a "toxic" impact on us. It is not that either person deliberately intends us good or harm, or that either is a particularly good or bad person; it is simply an effect they have on us. It probably has a lot to do with how we related to our parents at a very young age. Many people have one parent who seems accepting and nurturing, no matter what we do, and with whom we always feel good, while the other parent is more critical and demanding and negative. Both may love us equally, but they simply have a different style. It may be that people who remind us of our nurturing parent make us feel good, and vice versa. "Well", you might say, "wouldn't people then always go for the people who are nurturing for them in friends, spouses and colleagues?" Surprisingly, this is often not the case. It may well be that the parent who is most toxic is the one whom you respect the most and many people end up marrying those toxic people. You are used to the critical destructive behaviour and it does not feel unusual to you.

Well, if you recognise these patterns in your life, and most people do, what can you do about it? We do not suggest you divorce your wife if you find her toxic, resign your job if you find your boss toxic or kick your toxic children out of the house. The first thing you can do is to be aware of this phenomenon. Just knowing that this can and is happening will enable you to create a distance in your mind between what is happening and the effect it has on you. Several people on these weekends have told us that this realisation is the single most important concept they get out of the weekend. Just realising that that is why your mother-in-law always irritates you can be very helpful.

But, as a cancer patient, you do have a certain extra power. You can identify those friends who are nurturing and those who are toxic. If you want to avoid someone you can be "tired", or "ill" or need to sleep. You can make excuses with those people and encourage those people who are nurturing in your life. Surround yourself with more nurturing people and the quality of your relationships will automatically increase.

What do you do about those people who are toxic, apart from creating distance? That is a very difficult question. In reality it is very difficult to change the relationship. Being aware of the nature of the relationship may itself make it easier, but the feelings involved may be very powerful. It may be more practical to encourage those who are nurturing and gently discourage those people who have a negative effect on you.

**Cancer – what is it, what can be done about it now and what possibilities might be available in the future?**

*Maurice:* Many of you might know quite a lot about cancer and its treatment, but I thought that before looking at what possibilities may come up in the future, it would be important to put them in the perspective of what we know about cancer now, and what treatments are used at the moment. The main thing about cancer is that there is a production of new cells which happens in an uncontrolled way. The body is made of billions of cells. If you cut your hand, the cells that are immediately next to that cut start dividing and produce new cells to fill the gap. As soon as the gap is filled the cells stop dividing and switch off. So they somehow know that they need so many million cells to fill the gap and as soon as that job is done, they stop reproducing themselves. So there is a form of control over how many of them are produced. What happens with cancer is that for some reason a cell gets switched on to produce more cells without any obvious reason to do so, without any hole to repair or damage to correct. So, if a cell starts dividing on the back of your hand, after a while a lot of new cells will have been produced. It goes quickly from two cells to four, eight, sixteen, thirty-two, sixty-four and so on. Eventually a lump will form on the back of the hand. The lump is the first problem with any cancer. If the lump is on the back of the hand it's not likely to cause much problem except cosmetically. But you could have a lump in a part of the body where it might block a tube or press against a nerve or damage a bone and therefore cause some pain or damage. The lump is, however, only a part of the problem. The thing that makes cancer dangerous is that some of the cells are able to get into the blood vessels and via these blood vessels can travel to other parts of the body. So, for example, a few cells might settle in the liver, some could settle in the lung, and some could settle in the brain. Now these cells have the capacity to divide and produce new cells so that the one cell that settles out in the liver could eventually produce a lump consisting of millions of cells. And similarly, the cells that have settled out in the lung and those in the brain can also form lumps there. These are known as secondaries or metastases.

Now, if we come back to the treatment for cancer, the first treatment which is usually considered by the doctor is surgery. Now why surgery? In the early stages of any cancer it will only be in one spot. If you are able to catch the cancer while it's still in one place then removing the cancer will by definition have cured it. But you might say "Ah well, that's what you say, but I know a person who has had a breast lump removed and the doctors told her it was all clear and yet years later she developed cancer in the liver and the lungs or the bones," and so on. This is absolutely true and this does happen. Cancer cells are very small. You can in fact get about ten thousand of them on the head of a pin. And the scans that we've got are not able to detect a lump if it's much smaller than the nail on your little finger. And a lump this size actually contains many millions of cells, so the only way we can know what the likelihood is of somebody being cured after any particular operation is from our past experience of what happens to patients with that type of tumour. In some cases we might expect that 90 per cent of people with this cancer will never come back. In other words, in 90 per cent of people it will not have spread at the time of the operation. In other cases there may be a very great risk that the cancer will come back because it is likely to have spread, even though we can't detect the cancer anywhere else in the body. So surgery is often an excellent treatment for cancer, in fact often the best treatment for cancer that hasn't spread to other parts of the body. Unfortunately, in many cases, the cancer has already spread at the time of diagnosis.

Another major treatment for cancer which many of you have had is radiotherapy. Radiotherapy consists of shining various sorts of rays on a part of the body which has the cancer. These rays are capable of destroying the cancer cells. They also damage the cells around the tumour, although with modern radiotherapy using computers, it is now possible to focus the rays very accurately so that they concentrate mostly on the cancer and very little on the normal tissues. But radiotherapy does cause some damage to normal tissues and there is a limit to how much you can actually use on any particular part of the body. For example, if you've got a single lump in the lung, you may be able to give a lot of radiotherapy to that lump with the aim of destroying it completely and accept the fact that you will destroy a bit of the surrounding lung. We've got two lungs and lots of spare lung capacity, so you can afford to do that. On the other hand, if you've got several spots of cancer throughout the lungs it becomes impossible to get rid of them with radiotherapy without destroying too much of the normal lung. So radiotherapy is a little bit like surgery in many ways. If you're using it to try and cure someone, you can only really do that if there is cancer in just one place. Sometimes radiotherapy can be used instead of surgery and I'll discuss this in more detail when we talk about the advances that have taken place in surgery and radiotherapy in a little while. But a good example is in the early stages of cancer of the larynx, which is cancer of the voice box. It can be treated by removing the voice box with surgery. This is a major operation which leaves a person having to speak through a hole in the bottom of their throat and has a very major effect on their lives. Alternatively, it can be treated with radiotherapy which causes very few side effects and the results are exactly the same. So clearly there is little doubt what option will be better in those circumstances. Similarly, if a cancer is in the brain and it is impossible to remove it with an operation without causing major permanent damage to the brain, then it may be better to treat it with radiotherapy. The other very useful place for radiotherapy is for the control of symptoms such as pain. A very small amount of radiotherapy to a particularly painful spot of cancer, say in the bones, can cause dramatic relief with very few side effects from the radiotherapy. Similarly, if someone is coughing up blood because of a lung cancer, a little bit of radiotherapy to that spot can relieve the symptoms very effectively with few side effects.

The other treatment for cancer is drug treatment. Drug treatment has a number of theoretical advantages over radiotherapy and surgery because drugs get into the blood stream and via the blood stream are distributed all over the body. So if you've got cancer cells in the liver or the lungs or the bones the drugs can get there because they go to all parts of the body. It is similar to treating an infection with antibiotics. The antibiotics will get in the blood stream and will be able to kill the germs wherever they are in the body. There are two different sort of drugs which are used. The first is hormone therapy. There are some tumours such as breast cancer and cancer of the prostate which will often respond to these hormonal treatments. The other drug treatment is chemotherapy and I'm going to talk a little bit more about chemotherapy.

Chemotherapy is a group of drugs that kill cancer cells. Unfortunately, they also damage some normal cells in the body. There has been a lot of publicity in the press about the side effects of chemotherapy. Many people think of chemotherapy as one thing and that all chemotherapy is the same. Now first of all this is a mistake. Chemotherapy ranges from treatment which consists of a few tablets every month which cause very few side effects to intensive therapy, which can cause lots of side effects. Now how does chemotherapy work? As I've just said, chemotherapy doesn't only damage the cancer cells, it also damages the normal cells. As everybody here who has received chemotherapy knows, what usually happens is that you get it in a day or a few days, followed by a rest period. The reason for this is that although chemotherapy damages both the normal cells and the cancer cells, the normal cells recover very quickly from the damage whilst the cancer cells recover very slowly. So if, for example, you give chemotherapy today and you damage both the normal cells and the cancer cells, in 3 weeks' time the normal cells will have recovered but the cancer cells will still be damaged. So you treat again. You further damage the cancer cells but the normal cells will recover again after a 3-week rest. This can be repeated and you progressively damage the cancer cells but do not cause progressive damage to the normal cells. Chemotherapy doesn't work in all cancers. In some cancers it can be given even in very advanced stages with good chance of cure. And those are the cancers where it is used very intensively and where doctors and patients feel that the side effects are acceptable in exchange for the possibility of being cured. It is always difficult to know who will be cured and who will not; some people have the chemotherapy and don't benefit and that's a very difficult situation for both doctors and patients. There are other situations where you know that chemotherapy may shrink the cancer, but is unlikely to make it go away completely. The treatment is therefore given to relieve symptoms and to prolong life. In those circumstances we would use much milder chemotherapy. Chemotherapy which, if possible, doesn't make you very sick or take your hair out and which certainly doesn't suppress your blood count to the point where it is dangerous. What your doctor will suggest in terms of chemotherapy depends to a large extent on what he believes he can realistically hope to achieve with the treatment, as well as what you want and what you are prepared to accept.

Now there is another situation which I think I should mention because many people here have had breast cancer, and that is the situation of adjuvant drug treatment either with hormone treatment or chemotherapy. Adjuvant treatment means treatment in addition to surgery. You will remember that I mentioned that in some patients the doctor knows that even if the operation removes all the visible cancer, there is a very good chance of it coming back. We only know that because of our past experience of that particular type and stage of cancer. Under those circumstances, why wait until such time as the cancer comes back? We know that cancer is much easier to treat and cure if it's treated very early, even with chemotherapy. So why not give the drug treatment immediately after surgery? This adjuvant therapy is used mostly for some patients with breast cancer and bowel cancer, and for some children's cancers, as well as some other cancers.

What have been the advances in the treatment of cancer over the past few years? Chemotherapy first became available in its modern form about 20 years ago. There were major advances in the treatment of patients with conditions like Hodgkin's disease and non-Hodgkin's lymphomas, and several of the children's tumours became curable for the first time, even when these cancers were advanced. In the mid-1970s with the development of a new drug called cisplatinum, testicular cancer (you may be surprised to hear that this is the commonest cancer in young men) suddenly became curable in the majority of patients, whereas before most patients died of this disease. There have been some pretty dramatic developments, though most improvements in cancer treatment happen in small stages, bit by bit. There are many small improvements which are taking place all the time, which are too detailed and numerous to go into here. Cancer treatment is also becoming more sophisticated. By combining surgery and radiotherapy it is now often possible in patients with breast cancer not to have to remove the breast. The lump is taken out and radiotherapy given to the breast leaving the woman with a breast that is similar cosmetically to the other breast. It is now possible in many more patients who have cancer of the rectum not to have to remove the lower part of the rectum and the anus, but to rejoin the bowel after removing the cancer and obviously that's a great advantage. Because of this more people can avoid having a colostomy (a "bag"). Similarly, in people who have cancer of the arm or leg (called sarcomas), it is now often possible to remove only the lump or the bit of bone that is involved and then give radiotherapy to destroy any remaining cancer. The person has just as good a chance of survival as with the removal of the arm or leg. As you know, one of the major side effects with chemotherapy is nausea and vomiting. Over the past few years drugs to combat the nausea and vomiting have been developed, which are much more successful at treating it, compared to a few years ago. Even though these developments might not sound very dramatic, they are certainly very important from the point of view of both the patient receiving the treatment and the doctor giving it. More recently, a substance has been produced by genetic engineering which may well be able to reduce significantly the amount that chemotherapy reduces the cells in the bone marrow and the blood, thereby reducing the most dangerous aspect of intensive chemotherapy.

What about the future? Well, let's first of all look at the available treatments. First, surgery and radiotherapy. Surgery as a treatment for cancer is clearly limited because the major problem with cancer is that it spreads to other parts of the body. It is not possible to do hundreds of operations however good the operations. So surgical techniques will improve so that the operations cause less problems for the patients, but it's unlikely that improvements in surgical technique will dramatically improve the cure rate for cancer. The same thing applies to radiotherapy. Radiotherapy will continue to improve by using techniques that enable the radiotherapy to focus more closely on the tumour. Using computers to outline the tumour, it will be possible to cause less and less damage to normal tissues, but radiotherapy can only be given to a limited amount of the body and so it is unlikely that further developments in radiotherapy are going to make a difference between curing somebody or not curing them. The place where major advances are going to come in the future in the treatment of cancer is with drug treatment. There are a number of different ways these are likely to come about. New research is going on in the laboratory and with animals all the time to investigate new hormone drugs and new chemotherapy agents. There have been a number of times in the past 15 years where this line of research has led to dramatic improvements, as I've already mentioned when I referred to the drug cisplatinum in the case of testicular cancer. At the same time, research is carrying on with the current drugs to reduce their side effects. For example, we now have drugs for some cancers which cause very little nausea and don't cause hair loss, which are as effective as the older drugs. The next line of research is into a totally new group of drugs which in the broadest sense of the word are called biological response modifiers. That means that these are natural substances which are produced by the body in tiny amounts in the normal course of events to help you fight infection and cancer. By genetic engineering it is now possible to produce them in very large amounts so they can actually be used as drugs. There are many of these agents which are being tested at the moment. They include substances like interferon, tumour necrosis factor, interleuken and so on. A lot of work is needed to know whether or not this new group of drugs is going to be helpful. We already know, for example, that interferon can be very useful in some patients with a rare type of leukaemia called hairy cell leukaemia and possibly in chronic myeloid leukaemia and an unusual type of cancer called carcinoid tumour. The substances I mentioned earlier which prevent the reduction of the blood count and the cells in the bone marrow by chemotherapy are also biological response modifiers. These may enable doctors to give bigger and more effective doses of chemotherapy than previously and might result in an improvement in treatment.

Research is also going on to try and understand what it is that makes cancer cells grow in an uncontrolled fashion. Evidence is now available which suggests that this may well be due to the production of growth factors by the cells themselves. Research is now going on to try and look at possible drugs which would be able to switch off these growth factors and by that means switch off the growth of the cancer. We could also ask, "What inside the cancer cell makes it produce these growth factors?" There is now quite a lot of information from research suggesting that in cancer cells a certain group of genes called oncogenes have become "switched on". It is these oncogenes which could possibly result in the production of the growth factors. So another way of tackling cancer in the future may be to develop drugs which switch the onco-genes off again.

Another way of tackling cancer is to try and make treatments which are directed against the cancer itself without going to the normal tissues, the so called "magic bullet" effect. This would have the advantage that only the cancer would be damaged and not the normal tissues. You could then give as much of the drug as you needed to kill the cancer. This could be achieved by using monoclonal antibodies. Antibodies are able to distinguish one tissue or one substance from another. We have them in our body all the time. For example, if you get chicken pox you don't usually get it again. This is because when you get another chicken pox virus entering the body, antibodies that were formed from the previous infection recognise the chicken pox virus and they kill it right away, before it can give you chicken pox. Now monoclonal antibodies are just a very pure form of these antibodies. They are developed against cancer cells and the idea is that you attach a small amount of radio-activity or a very poisonous drug to the monoclonal antibodies and when you give them to the patient they would go to the cancer and not the normal cells. People have been doing research on this for a number of years and we know that they work to some extent. The problem is that, although they go more to the cancer cells than to the normal tissues, they still go to normal tissues as well. So, for example, you might get five times as much of the monoclonal antibodies in the cancer cells as in the normal tissues. Unfortunately, we need much more in the cancer cells relative to normal tissues before they are able to cure cancer patients. For example, it may be necessary to have 40 or 50 times as much in the cancer cells compared to the normal tissues, but certainly the principle works to some extent and in the future it may be that this will be very useful for treating cancer patients.

Having mentioned all these things to you, I think I should say that one of the major things about research these days is that there is very rapid communication of new information. This takes place by means of computers, journals, and also with the many meetings around the world. As a result of all this, information is communicated very quickly from one doctor to another. So if research takes place in, say, South America, which made a big difference to the treatment of cancer, everybody in the field all around the world would know about it quite quickly. It is important to remember that even though many of these things are in the research phase, and haven't yet reached the point where they are being used to treat cancer patients successfully, any one of them might become successful and there may be a breakthrough at any time in the future. So the situation is never hopeless, even if at the moment the current treatments which are available for your cancer are not likely to be of benefit.

## CONCLUSION

The insights we obtained during these weekend seminars led us to the conclusion that the period after the discovery of cancer may provide someone with their greatest challenge, to make the best of every moment. Living each day with the possibility of death can help us negate our fear of it, we may even transcend this fear.

The next chapter describes the story of Vicky Clement Jones, whose name has already been mentioned during these weekend seminars as someone who resisted fear and defeat and lived each hour to the fullest.

She embodied many of the qualities people strive to achieve and that we hope the weekend seminars may stimulate.

# Chapter 3

# Vicky

*Nira:* On a sunny, Saturday morning in January 1986, Maurice and I were strolling in a park in Tel Aviv. Maurice was telling me about the creation of BACUP, the newly born Cancer Information Service, inspired and constructed by one of his patients, Dr Vicky Clement Jones. His story was about the service, since we were discussing the Maagalim Crisis Intervention Centre in Israel and comparing the services. Our chat touched time and time again on this patient of his, Vicky.

In the beginning I answered by saying it is not unusual for people coming out of their own crisis to have the need to save others from hardships, especially those that can be avoided. Maurice tried to tell me something I had heard many times before in my life as a therapist. He felt this person was special. The main reasons he gave for her specialness were: energy, brightness, leadership, enthusiasm and innovativeness in the way she started this organisation. And then he added that all this was in a young woman who had incurable cancer.

To me, at the time, cancer was bad enough and I could hardly visualise the difference between curable and incurable cancer, since both had the word "cancer" in them. I have come a long way since that morning. Not only has the word "cancer" a different meaning to death, but the name "Vicky Clement Jones" has become unique and special. On my next trip to London, Maurice initiated a meeting between Vicky and me. Vicky, through Maurice, had become interested in psychology and Maurice convinced her it would be interesting to have me work on her "lifestyle", trying to understand her basic motivations and patterns of personality. This was a rather awkward introduction and to this day I am not sure whether Vicky agreed to our meeting just to please her doctor.

We met at BACUP in a tiny room, almost a cubicle, in the midst of telephones ringing, computers hammering, people coming in and out and everything carrying the smell of "new paint" and pioneer spirit. Then Vicky came in. I was taken by surprise. Expecting "a grand lady", I met a child-like, frail girl, dressed in a jumper and skirt, with short hair, dancing eyes and – I later learned – several pipes and tubes from different parts of her body under her clothes. She certainly belonged to this place. She welcomed me and hurried me to the room where we were to talk.

Vicky regarded this as a "session". Very little time was wasted on introduction; she was eager to tell me her story and hear what I had to say. Up to this point, I hadn't experienced much real curiosity. I, too, had been pushed into this meeting by Maurice. Nor did I think our meeting would have any special meaning, other than my getting to know Vicky.

Four hours later, having listened and been involved in a vivid question and answer session, I did not feel any closer to Vicky than before, but I joined the group of people who could not express exactly why Vicky fascinated them, because above all her other skills, there was a strong sense of denial of death in its highest form, the one called heroism.

After Vicky had died and all the obituaries had been written and the grand memorial service had been held at St Paul's Cathedral, Maurice, who was her doctor, who had helped her set up BACUP and who was her close friend, shared with me his loss of both the person and the phenomenon.

It occurred to us that it is normal for people to write about their cancer, including describing the support of their doctors. It is much less common for doctors, who are first-hand witnesses to the struggle and the conquest, to write about cancer other than as case histories, to be published in medical journals, when it is as though the cancer has the person! So we have combined the story of Vicky, told by her doctor who influenced her and was influenced and inspired by her over the past 5 years, with the story told by Vicky herself from the transcripts of my interviews with her and her writings.

This story is not meant to be a memorial or an enlarged obituary. It is a story about a woman who tried to encourage people with cancer to discover their freedom and to use it in their own way. Professor McElwain said, "she was a star". We call people stars because we see them as a universe apart from us. Those rare people, like Vicky, who shine with knowledge even from an arm's length, are not simply stars, they are real people.

## FIRST ENCOUNTER

*Maurice:* When I first met Vicky she was a senior registrar at St Bartholomew's Hospital in the Department of Endocrinology. I don't think I had ever spoken to her before when I received a "yellow board" (a yellow piece of card from another consultant in the hospital asking you to see a new patient). It was from a professor of surgery and he asked me if I would see this Vicky Clement Jones. I had a busy afternoon and decided to set aside about three-quarters of an hour to go and see her. I was introduced to this small, attractive, Chinese woman who was 33 years old. She was in bed having just had an operation a couple of days before and was sitting up, very bright and quite cheerful. The first impression I had was that she was very welcoming and very enthusiastic. She had just been told she had cancer. I remember being surprised at how pleased she was to see me. Patients usually treat the first visit of a cancer doctor with great trepidation: "What is he going to tell me?" She almost appeared to divorce the situation from herself, and was eager to see this doctor who could tell her what she wanted to know. There was a degree of anxiety, but she didn't give me the impression she was depressed.

When I see a new patient I normally find out what has happened to them by taking their medical history. I then examine them and discuss my findings with the patient and usually the family as well. I spent a long time with Vicky, I think it was about 2 hours. Right from the very beginning she wanted to know all about her situation, what it meant, details about what they had found at the operation and all the types of treatment available. It was difficult for me to finish taking her history because she had so many questions to ask. In fact, she had already written down a long list of questions before I arrived and took notes of my answers. Vicky was so full of enthusiasm and questions, it was difficult to conduct the interview by the normal routine and schedule. She had her own schedule and it was more a case of her interviewing me, rather than my interviewing her.

When I see a patient for the first time, I am very much in control of the situation. I always try to judge how much information to give a patient at the first visit and how to present the information in a way that is honest, but does not remove hope. So there is a certain amount of editing of information, even when you are being open about the diagnosis and treatment of cancer. How much information I give depends on many things. Most importantly, how much the patient wants to know and how much he or she asks. An elderly lady, who is anxious and alone and asks few questions, may need to be given the information in stages, compared to a young woman who is well supported and demands all the information you have. I also try to involve patients in their own treatment decisions by giving them information so the decisions can ultimately come from them and their family. Some patients like this approach, others prefer the doctor to make all the decisions for them.

## DEALING WITH THE DIAGNOSIS

*Maurice:* With Vicky I certainly was not controlling the situation, even from the first interview. She was very respectful and obviously interested in what I was saying, but she was saying clearly: "This is my body and my life, and nobody makes decisions for me." From her history I found out that a year before her ovarian cancer was discovered, she had had appendicitis. When she developed the pain in her abdomen she was initially thought to have an abscess and was operated on with this in mind. No-one really suspected she had ovarian cancer. During the operation it became clear she had extensive cancer, which had spread beyond the ovaries throughout the lining of the abdomen. It was, in fact, inoperable. She had very advanced cancer.

In the very early stages of ovarian cancer it can be cured by operation alone. In the more advanced stages, however, it is treated with surgery and a combination of drugs, such as chemotherapy. Even in very advanced cases like Vicky's, a minority of women can, in fact, be cured with this treatment. The majority of people are not. Despite this, for many women, the treatment will shrink their cancer, relieve their symptoms and prolong their lives. Vicky had a small chance of the cancer being cured and a good chance of having temporary shrinkage of the cancer. I explained all this to her in detail. Normally when I talk to patients I tell them what is happening and what treatment they might receive, but I don't usually discuss statistics because I think in general it is not very helpful. Statistics apply to population and not to individuals and I try to explain that each person has an individual programme of treatment and no-one can predict accurately what will happen. Vicky was an unusual patient in that she wanted all the statistics and wrote them all down. I think her taking notes was an indication of her long-term planning, the methodological way she approached the illness. It really implied hope and determination. Although it was unusual for someone to want all the statistics and facts, I believe it is a person's right to know. I also had a strong feeling it was right for Vicky. It was what she clearly wanted and needed. I also knew, of course, when she had finished talking to me, she would go and read medical books and journals, so there was no point in bluffing her, not that I would have wanted to anyway.

I also suggested to Vicky she might find it useful to get a second opinion, to have somebody else with whom she could independently discuss her situation. I asked whether she wanted to see another colleague in London, or possibly even see somebody in the United States. She had told me her family had many connections there. She didn't want that at all.

I found Vicky's approach to her cancer stimulating and fascinating. I could not help admiring her courage and positive approach. I realised later that in some respects we had similar personalities, both being a bit "over the top" and overenthusiastic. You sometimes meet somebody and get on very well with them, right from the beginning – you "click". Vicky and I got on very well, very quickly, and became friends. There is no doubt if we had met in different circumstances, we would have been friends. If we had been working in the same department we would have worked quite well together. I found myself enjoying conversation with her. Often I go and see a new patient and, if I am feeling tired, I have to work up the energy to spend time with them and give them what they need. Talking to Vicky made me feel stimulated and, even though I was tired when I went to see her, and spent a long time talking to her, I enjoyed our conversation and felt challenged by her demanding behaviour.

When I used to see her regularly in the days that followed, telling her what was going on and planning the treatment, I always looked forward to our talks, despite the painful, difficult decisions we had to make. She gave me the impression she considered the information I gave her very carefully and it made a real difference to her. I felt it was important to her to have the information and she received it with great enthusiasm and vitality. It is very difficult to describe this magnetism; many people who met her when she was setting up BACUP noticed this same energy, enthusiasm and vitality and came away fully committed to her cause.

I found her whole approach to cancer stimulating and interesting. At the first interview she was setting the rules. In effect she was saying "You will have to work for me."

## DEALING WITH TREATMENT. GAINING CONTROL

*Vicky:* I had an inkling that it might be cancer when I was coming round from the anaesthetic. I asked the houseman whether it was an appendix abscess. He said it wasn't an abscess and the professor would come and see me tomorrow. So he was saying I had something very, very serious, but I was groggy at the time. I thought "This will go away, I am sure it's a dream. I will wake up and it's all not true." There was no evidence other than what the houseman had said that I had anything serious. The next morning the senior registrar (a more senior doctor) came to see me. He had a gloomy stance, the way people behave when you can tell they are bringing you bad news. He drew the curtains round and said that when they had looked into my abdomen it wasn't an abscess. They had taken a small bit of tissue from the abdomen and he told me what they saw. I am not even sure he used the word "cancer". I felt, "This is not happening to me." It just felt unreal. The ward was bustling and cheerful. I had been ill twice the year before and I thought how unfair it was. Somehow, from the first moment I was told I had cancer, I felt like a different person. The first thing I felt was, "Why me?" and I felt guilty. I was brought up as a Roman Catholic and I had become a lapsed Roman Catholic. I somehow felt my three illnesses were a punishment, but then I thought, I have been doing all the right things, what had I done that was so bad? So I thought a lot about guilt, punishment and "Why me?" and that night I threw religion out of the window. It was like stopping the game, a child's game like Ludo, or Monopoly. I decided to opt out of the game altogether so there could be no more problems. I closed the book and said, "Right, that's it – I've had three illnesses and I'm going to try something else." That something else was believing in myself. I discovered that felt right and it made me feel good to believe in myself. Maybe I had never believed in myself before. At school, even though I was very bright, I was very frightened of failing, that I wouldn't come up to the mark.

That afternoon Maurice came to see me, being the cancer doctor at Bart's specialising in cancer of the ovary. I hadn't met him before because he was a young doctor who had only recently been appointed a consultant. I had, in fact, just written to him to refer a patient, and had then seen his name for the first time. I very much enjoyed our first conversation. We are both quite manic in that we talk very quickly. The two of us talked manically for an hour, or two. Intellectually we were very similar. We fired on each other and I felt a bond was formed, even at that point. I was a little older than him and I thought the news he brought was incredible; the fact that there was some treatment for cancer of the ovary. In many ways the news was not very optimistic, but at least there was some hope. I didn't have confidence the treatment would work, but I had great confidence in Maurice. Before he came I felt I had been in a shipwreck and I was clinging to a raft, getting colder and colder, beginning to give up hope and thinking I was going to drown at any time. Maurice came like a knight on a white charger, but in a boat, saving me from drowning.

He told me I would need 3 months of intensive chemotherapy, which had many side effects and then, if the cancer responded well, it may be possible for the surgeons to operate again, to try to remove the disease. So over the next few days I decided in those 3 months I was going to concentrate on being happy, doing things that made me happy and surrounding myself with things that would be happy. My prime aim was to enjoy myself, treat myself to happiness, not work hard and just see how it went.

*Maurice:* I explained to Vicky she needed chemotherapy to treat her cancer. These are anti-cancer drugs that travel the blood stream and can therefore reach cancer anywhere in the body. The problem with these drugs is they can have many side effects. Vicky was given three drugs at the same time. They were given to her once a month by injection into a vein. They made her quite sick for a few days and caused her hair to fall out. They also temporarily caused a decrease in the number of blood cells in her blood. This meant she had to be admitted to hospital for a few days every month for treatment with drips, blood transfusions and antibiotics. After 3 chemotherapy treatments, 3 months later, we did a scan of her abdomen and pelvis. It was obvious from the scan the disease had shrunk quite dramatically and it looked as though it might be possible to carry out an operation. At the operation most of the disease was removed. This was a great improvement on the first operation when it had not been possible to remove anything. There were, though, several small nodules of cancer left behind, so she had another three chemotherapy treatments and, 3 months later, yet another operation. At this third operation it appeared all the disease had disappeared. There was actually nothing to see that was abnormal at all. Despite this, the surgeon took many tiny pieces of tissue (called biopsies) from about 30 different places in her abdomen. When these were examined under the microscope, it showed a few of them still had tiny amounts of ovarian cancer left. This was very vital information because even though the disease was now very small, and over 99 per cent of the ovarian cancer had been destroyed, we knew that if left unchecked, cancer would grow back again. So she had further chemotherapy with different drugs in an attempt to get rid of the remaining small amount of cancer. Her disease was very sensitive to chemotherapy, but there was no way of knowing if she had been given enough. Only by waiting to see whether the disease came back would we know the final outcome.

This was a very frustrating, anxious time for Vicky and her husband Tim. At every stage Vicky asked to be given information to think about it. She needed to discuss it with Tim and, on a number of occasions, asked me to talk separately to him and other members of the family. In the beginning she was very keen to read medical journals herself. She used to say, "I've read this, what does this mean? How does this fit in with what you say?" "Somebody else in this journal says he does things slightly differently, why are you doing what you are doing?" This wasn't done to catch me out, it was just her way of coping. She needed to know why everything was happening to her. After a while she stopped reading so intensively, but in the first few months she went through a period of reading everything she could get her hands on. There was a strange paradox in Vicky's search for information. For many people denial is a way of coping. For others information seeking, a compulsive need for knowledge, is the way they deal with critical situations. While Vicky clearly was an extreme example of the latter, she also strongly denied the possibility of death at an emotional level. She discussed it logically, as if she was talking about someone else, but did not relate it to herself. Vicky had to know the reasons behind everything being done to her, the rationale and the chances of success. She felt at every point she made her own decisions and was completely in control. I always encourage patients to be involved in decision making but, in reality, most of them base their decision largely on what the doctor advises. That is, of course, completely reasonable as the doctor is the expert with the most information. Vicky considered my advice very carefully, but most of the decisions were made by her. She was completely in control and I sometimes felt she was using me simply to get information.

That was just one side of it. She also saw the doctor as someone who was working with her to help herself get better. She had a strong feeling of equality and partnership. This partnership could not be on quite the same basis if the patient were not a doctor. I love teaching. With patients like Vicky I feel the way I do when I have highly intelligent, appreciative students. They are fun to teach and I learn from them. I have had several other patients who adopt a very similar attitude to Vicky. The only difference is, they were more dependent on me for information. Vicky was also more extreme than most people in her desire to be sure she understood correctly. What Vicky and these other patients do is challenge their doctor in an intelligent, involved way. It did not feel demanding or draining. I should add, Vicky was not an easy patient by any means and I would not be able to cope with too many "Vickys" at the same time! Not only would she spend a long time with me in the hospital, but she would frequently telephone me at home. At times when she was having difficulties I would expect at least one telephone call a night, sometimes more. She would ring to discuss things and go over them again and again to make sure she understood. In many ways this was completely over the top and I have never given another patient so much of my time, either before or after Vicky. She made herself exceptional because of her hard work and intelligent involvement in her illness. I respected her for that. She may have given the impression she was preoccupied with her illness and, in a way, she was. She was, however, not very anxious; she simply saw her illness as a project and was concerned she got it exactly right. She took the same logical approach to her illness as to a problem with her research in the laboratory.

There was no doubt this was a very unusual relationship between a doctor and a patient. I enjoyed talking to her; she stimulated me and I found her interesting. I somehow never felt threatened by her, even though she questioned everything I did and I had to justify every statement I made. I felt she trusted me. She had always read the journals before me. If the journals came out on Monday, she had read the relevant articles by Monday night, while it usually took me a few weeks to get round to reading them. In the beginning, when she started doing that, I used to feel a bit irritated. She would even have the papers delivered to my secretary the very day they came out, to make sure I had read them in time for her to ask me about them.

At the point when Vicky completed her chemotherapy and operations, I had to explain it was impossible to know whether there was any cancer left and there was a possibility the cancer might come back. Vicky always took the most positive attitude, so she decided she was going to regard herself as "cured". She was going to live a normal life from then on.

## A SECOND LOOK AT LIFE

*Maurice:* What was unusual about Vicky was not that she had been through that sort of treatment. Many others do too. What was unusual was the courageous way she faced up to problems; the direct way she dealt with them. The chances of living, or dying, the side effects and so on. I really admired her courage to go on living a nearly normal life, not giving up her fun and joys. She expected to enjoy life and did not ask for any sympathy or special treatment. I think that requires a special attitude and courage. Vicky would say she had learnt to appreciate difficulties her patients had and she saw herself becoming a better doctor as a result. She had learnt to appreciate what it was like to be well and felt being faced with serious illness gave her strength and courage to use later in life. She believed, on a personal and philosophical level, she was learning about life and about struggling. She spoke about cancer changing her from a future-orientated to a present-orientated person. Many people comment how cancer taught them to "live in the present" and learn how to live "now". Once she was sick and had acknowledged the concept of death, if only briefly, she realised how important it was to have fun.

In the beginning, I had difficulty deciding how to balance our doctor/patient relationship with our friendship. As a doctor you have to talk to people about a very personal side of their lives. Doctors have to examine people, for example, which can be embarrassing for the person concerned and is much easier if the doctor is distant from them. It may be important they don't see the doctor as a real person, but someone to whom they don't relate, as it would be too embarrassing for them. For doctors, too, it is easier to remain at a distance for similar reasons. As a young doctor I initially felt awkward and embarrassed talking to patients intimately and doing internal examinations. I gradually learnt to relax and feel at ease in these situations, but it is still much more awkward if I know someone well outside the clinic. The other point is, many patients say how important it is to look up to and respect their doctor. I don't think everyone would be encouraged in their relationship with their doctor to see him or her, for example, having fun at a party. I think people would rather see the doctor as a serious person, concerned about people being ill and would prefer not to see him or her as a whole person. I think most patients prefer a formal, but friendly relationship and complain about doctors who are over-familiar. You can achieve a balance between maintaining some distance from your doctor, someone who is not in any way personally connected with you, but still feel he or she cares about you and is actively involved in your treatment at every level. So there is a paradox between developing a relatively egalitarian relationship and giving people as much information as they want, and still allowing people to maintain their fantasy about their doctor.

It may seem Vicky broke this barrier and did not conform to the rules. However, this was not so. For example, when she came to the clinic to see me, we had clear rules which we had actually discussed. The first was we would not talk about anything other than her illness and I would regard her entirely as a patient until the consultation was completely finished. She would often want to rush ahead and talk about other things, but knew I wasn't prepared to talk to her about anything else until I had completed the process of asking how she was, examining her and discussing aspects related to her treatment and illness. When that was clearly finished, we would chat about other things. She would say it was almost like playing roles, but even though it was, we still did it every single time. Despite these rules I still felt awkward about being so friendly with a patient. I felt I was breaking the rules I had been taught throughout my training, rules which exist for good reasons. But then I realised Vicky was exceptional and this was an unusual doctor/patient relationship. I basically believed I should break the rules in this situation as it was clear she needed her doctor to work with her as part of a team and I enjoyed the relationship. I also must admit I identified with Vicky more than with other patients. She was a doctor, a colleague of a similar age, at a similar stage in her career, who had developed cancer. I frequently thought to myself, I would never have the courage to face cancer in the way she had. Undoubtedly I admired her and respected the way that she dealt with such overwhelming difficulties. I would have felt frightened to be in the same situation as Vicky was in and her courage was inspirational.

Vicky talked to me about what she should do with her life. She did not want to go back into endocrinology. She realised now that being in a laboratory would achieve very little. She felt she would be trying to "push back the frontiers of science by thumbnail". She said if she spent her whole life doing that, her contribution would be very small and not very personal. She felt she wanted to do something more related to cancer patients. The first thing she considered was to retrain as an oncologist. She talked to me very seriously about this. I dissuaded her. I felt it was a bad idea because to become involved in treating cancer patients would take 4 to 5 years of further study at least and she had a very high risk of the disease coming back. I also thought she might become too involved with cancer. I don't know if I was right or wrong, but that was the advice I gave her at the time. At any rate, I believed Vicky would do what felt right for her and my advice was only one factor she would consider. The other possibility she considered was to train as a GP. She felt she had a contribution to make and didn't want to waste her unique experience. Eventually she did decide to do general practice, possibly with a special interest in cancer and she hoped to have a job later in the cancer department as a clinical assistant. She signed up for a general practice training scheme. It was a tremendously difficult move for her as she was changing from an ambitious academic career to one where she could make a contribution to patients at a more personal level. She was very depressed during that time.

This is not uncommon when people finish cancer treatment. They go home and imagine they should feel elated because the treatment is over. I usually tell people at the end of treatment that although they anticipate they will feel elated, they are more likely to feel depressed. People are always surprised by the depression. They realise how dependent they have become on the regular visits to the hospital and how the treatment, however difficult, adds structure and security to their lives. Also, during the treatment, they are able to live from one visit to hospital to the next, and set short-term goals of getting through each treatment. Suddenly, when the treatment is over, they look at the rest of their lives and face up to the reality of cancer, perhaps for the first time. For the patient this has several components. You realise that although treatment is over, the cancer may not be; you may still have cancer or there is still the possibility it may recur. Beyond this, you find cancer has changed your life in other ways. Many people find life seems to have little meaning and purpose. The trauma of the diagnosis and treatment has resulted in a reappraisal of life and the old meaning and purpose have gone. It feels as though you are living in a vacuum. For many people this is a time of introspection, where they try to sort out the new meaning and their role in a new world. So the depression has a purpose and is often a time of change and growth. It is also a difficult time for family and friends who, by now, are exhausted and hope life can get back to normal, finding instead, life will never be normal again.

*Vicky:* The time I was most depressed was after the initial treatment finished and Maurice said, "You can go back to work." I had spent all my time struggling and focusing on staying alive and it was very difficult to refocus on anything new. I had not only been trying to stay alive, I had also worked hard at enjoying myself while going through all the treatments. Suddenly I didn't have the challenge of the treatments, going to hospital and seeing Maurice. People said I needed to reinvest in life and think of the future. But how could I reinvest in life when it was so uncertain? I might have a recurrence next week. More than that, I was depressed about my career. Somehow my high-powered research career had completely lost meaning. I thought, "I just can't do this any more."

Part of the depression was feeling there was no meaning in life. I wondered about my worth. Maybe I had been saved, but what for? What can I do? I wished I could be dead several times, although I never did anything about it. I had to get myself out of the depression. I used to write down what I was feeling; I used to write notes to myself and say to myself, "You know Vicky, this is ridiculous. Why are you doing this to yourself? Why are you so depressed? Shake yourself out of it." I came out of the depression about Christmas time when I started visiting GP practices to think about a new career to include cancer. I could be a GP and also do something in relation to cancer. I remember over the next 6 months while I was still working out what I was going to do, I went to a conference on cancer. I met other people. Maurice was there, and I found it all very exciting and challenging. I started feeling it was a new life. I could go into something and do something.

## ORDER AFTER CHAOS : THE START OF BACUP

*Maurice:* The first I heard about Vicky's idea of a cancer information service was some months after she had finished treatment. The idea was based on her experience in hospital, when patients used to come to her bedside to talk to her about cancer and ask questions again and again. In our department we tell people what is going on and much time is spent with people talking about cancer, not just by the consultant, but by junior doctors, nurses, social workers and other people. There is an openness about cancer, but despite that, Vicky found people used to come and ask her, seemingly for confirmation or reassurance, the same questions they had already asked their doctor and nurse. She wondered why they came to see her. Perhaps because she was a nice, approachable person, who explained things clearly. Perhaps because she was a doctor who would have accurate information. She felt, however, none of these really answered the question. One of her big insights was realising patients needed to talk to her, not just because she was who she was, but because they needed to talk to someone other than their doctor, who had information of an authoritative nature. And they wanted to do this again and again. From this she developed the idea of a cancer information service and came to see me about it. Right from the very beginning I thought it was an excellent idea and decided to back her. I was amazed people like myself, who had been looking after cancer patients for years, had not come up with this idea before. It was so obvious, so logical. Why had it required Vicky to think of it? She was enormously enthusiastic. She had been discouraged by not going into oncology and this gave her an opportunity to become directly involved in the field of cancer. From here on our relationship also changed. She now had her own role in the fight against cancer and we became more colleagues than doctor and patient.

I had misgivings about whether it was possible to get a cancer information service off the ground in this country. In the beginning I thought it might be difficult to get my medical colleagues to go along with it. Doctors in England tend to be conservative and their right to provide all the information they believe their patients need is carefully guarded. In the United States, where a cancer information service already existed, there had been considerable consumer pressure to provide this facility. In fact, the American National Cancer Institute provided the cancer information service at the instruction of Congress.

Initially I gave Vicky some introductions and suggested she met the major figures in the oncological establishment and the various support services. One of her greatest assets was her ability to win people over to her views. She also had a number of advantages, especially when talking to the medical profession. First, she was a doctor and second, anyone who saw her curriculum vitae realised she was a successful academic doctor. She had been a senior registrar at St Bartholomew's Hospital which, in itself, conveys an understanding that she was competent at her job, and her C.V. showed she had published her work quite extensively and was on her way to a successful academic career. She wrote to doctors, sending them a copy of her C.V. They then realised they were not just dealing with a patient with an idea, but with a doctor whom they could respect on equal terms. She had credibility, but more than that she was a patient. She could speak to doctors both as a colleague and patient. Her charisma was her major asset. She was enthusiastic, clearly spoken, and even though she was very ambitious, she never came across as threatening. People instantly liked her and saw her as an asset, not as competition. I am not sure quite why that was, because it certainly wasn't the situation in her past. Maybe the fact she was a patient removed some of the element of competitiveness she would otherwise have had if she had just been a doctor trying to set up an advisory service.

She managed to win over the support and enthusiasm of the oncologists in this country by going straight to the top; contacting the leading oncologists and getting them to agree to her idea. I think this was probably her biggest, single achievement. It is interesting that, in contrast to her overwhelming success with cancer specialists, she had more difficulty convincing her closest friends who, themselves, were doctors. There were many reasons for this; on the one hand, being doctors, they were nervous that it would be very difficult for something like this to succeed, but more than that they were concerned about whether it was the right thing for Vicky at this stage. She had just finished treatment and they felt she needed to take life easier, rest more and be kinder to herself. In addition, these close friends had spent the past year thinking and talking of nothing else other than Vicky's cancer. The time had come when they wanted to forget about cancer and return to a normal social existence, now that she was apparently well. This is a common paradox within families of cancer patients. When the patient has finished treatment the family want the patient to rest and help themselves to get better. In many ways, this is the last thing the patient wants. They need to get back to an active role in life, with new challenges and goals and are often more enthusiastic and energetic than ever before they became ill.

*Vicky:* I understood the concern of my friends that if I embarked on this project I might overdo things and not help my own health. They said many times – "But it's so much work" – and perhaps in their heart of hearts they felt it would be better for me to leave it to someone else. "Why not enjoy life", they said.

I believed I had been remarkably lucky to have survived to this point – I felt the experience I gained both medically and personally, maybe from an unusual perspective as both patient and doctor, coupled with my basic personality, enthusiasm and drive, might make the venture a reality. My illness changed my perspective on life. Returning to work at Bart's – being depressed and eventually deciding to leave academic medicine and go into general practice – is all part of this. I knew from the start, however, that giving up endocrinology and research and taking up general practice was something I really wanted to do because it involved patients as people and families – rather than as a walking store of "hormones" and "peptides". Although as an endocrinologist one may be very caring and work hard at the clinical side – the "buzz" comes from the research side – as do the rewards – which in academic medicine has to do with research papers and, ultimately, power. In that game you need to be out for yourself and personal advancement and, as Tim said, I'm not good at looking out for myself or personal gain. On the other hand, Tim always said I was good at fighting for causes and for others. Thus I came to the patient's organisation. One thing about it was I *really believed* in it – probably more than anything I had ever done before. What about the question – "Why not leave it for someone else to do?" With my medical and research background, as well as my experience as a patient, I found I had the skills to talk to people at many levels and reach them. In no sense did I feel I was the only one who could do it, it was not an ego trip. I gladly welcomed others who stepped forward and I actively sought such people as the task would have been impossible alone. Speaking to a number of people who know about the history of setting up charities, many said I was the one who should do it – and without me the project would fail. This again was not said to boost my sense of self-importance, but because I had the power of persuasion since my illness and my track record in many ways groomed me for the job.

I knew it would involve an incredible amount of work and there was a personal cost. I was very fortunate Tim is the person he is and believes in working for one's ideals. I could not be like him and work for 10 years for the Streatham Liberal Party, knocking on doors and getting the council to fix the windows and pavements for people. Moving forward so little towards his goal (at least in my eyes). I believed in the idea and I believed it should work. If you do not have a dream, it will never come true. I knew it was a dream, and a rather grand dream at that – but I was convinced it was possible and left no stone unturned in search of advice, funds, etc., to make it a reality.

As to the personal sacrifice, Tim also believed in the dream and, because of his civic nature, believes one should work for the ideal itself and not particularly for any material or other gain. I was very fortunate he was behind me and helped me tremendously. He knew it would mean me going to meetings, being busy on the phone, doing letters, but he understood this disruption of home life as he'd been doing the same for many years!

Another important point was I actually really enjoyed what I was doing. I believed in it, because I like talking to people about my ideas, and the rewards in terms of how you can help cancer patients and their families are incredible. I was doing something for myself and fulfilling the need to help others. Life is about choices – it was possible my ovarian cancer could come back at any time, so I did not feel I would be wasting my time and overdoing things, when I should be relaxing, sitting back and enjoying life.

It was a lonely task when I was "self-starting" – picking up the phone for the umpteenth time to try to get others interested, to ease the load, dictating sympathetic and articulate letters, going to meetings day after day on my own – and also knowing that, despite my experience, I needed to learn about administrative and management skills, as "the buck stopped here". It was my idea and wouldn't materialise without my striving. Don't think the prospect was not daunting, it was a question of drawing the strands together and keeping all the balls up in the air at the same time.

I knew I would not be satisfied in the long run if I worked quietly as a GP and did nothing else. I went into general practice to give myself mental space – what for, I did not know then – but I knew I wanted to work in support groups or something along that line – and this project was just an extension of that need. Some people said to me, "In your position, after what you've been through, I would want to forget about ever having cancer at all, start a new life and never talk about it again." Perhaps it was a burden on my friends as it reminded them all about my illness at a time when, having given me so much emotional support, they felt drained. In a way they would have preferred to forget about cancer altogether and just get on with living. David, one of my closest friends, had explained this point of view to me and I did understand. I also felt, however, that the needs of other patients and their families who were going through the experience now or in the future were just as important. In this sense, I was asking a lot of my friends.

My illness brought home to me the reality of my own mortality. I asked, "What are we in life for?" If I had a family with children or a husband who didn't understand why the project was important – I would not have dreamt of starting such a venture. Timmy, however, is the person he is and does public duty for whatever rewards he chooses – I think mainly because he feels it should be done and he has something to contribute. His experience and training, like my own, make him very suited to be the supportive husband of someone embarking on a venture like mine.

I felt well enough to take on the project – my only wish was I should stay well enough to get this dream started. I thought a personal sacrifice of 5 years to get it going was not too much for a project I believed in so much. I knew I might get ill in this time and not survive 5 years – but I did not think the time and energy would be wasted. Even at this early stage I had started to receive letters of thanks from people I had helped.

The key of a successful organisation is that, once going, it should be able to run without the boss. If, in 5 years' time, the service was up and running, it would not concern me if others took over – or if I were no longer here to see it happen – as long as the dream has been set in motion along the right tracks.

*Maurice:* The experience of cancer had clearly changed Vicky. Before she had cancer she was a hard-working, ambitious and talented doctor. She had not demonstrated any particular political or leadership skills, or had any interest in social projects. After the crisis she had been through, she used her highly developed organisational skills and talent as an innovator and combined them with new skills she had never known she possessed. I have no doubt, had she lived, she would not have gone back to medicine full-time, but would have developed very successfully in the medical/political arena. Although Vicky took the attitude she was cured, rather than wanting to get away from cancer, she did not want to waste her expertise and the special experience and insight she had gained. She felt if she didn't do something within the cancer field, much of what she had gained would be wasted. She also needed to find some meaning in what she had been through. If she could use her experience for the benefit of other people and make a contribution, she would have felt it was worthwhile. There is no doubt that, having had cancer, and being a patient, gave her new insight and new freedom. She no longer felt the necessity to succeed within the medical establishment. In the past she had a great desire to succeed and to impress her colleagues and superiors. She often talked about her need to impress her father. Once she had cancer she was somehow freed from this need and was prepared to be much more courageous and to go for something much less likely to bring her credit, especially in the academic world. Her decision to go into general practice shows how much her values had changed. Her desire to "push back the frontiers of science by a thumbnail" had now diminished. She wanted to make a contribution at a personal and social level.

Once she had decided to set up a cancer information service, and had the support of the oncology doctors, it was envisaged we would have a single oncology nurse answering the telephones. Even Vicky did not think very big in the beginning. We never thought as far as having secretaries and supporters. We certainly never thought of having a large set-up. We spent a long time agonizing about the name. We took a Saturday morning together going through ideas for the charity in my office at Bart's, then went for lunch at Simpsons in the Strand. This is a wonderful English restaurant, famous for roast beef. I didn't realise how formal it was; I arrived in denims and had to be lent a dinner jacket by the establishment. Vicky was engrossed in trying to find a name for this new organisation. She wanted something British and felt strongly it should be "A British Association of something". We tried to brainstorm what we wanted the charity to do and the name BACUP came to me in an inspired moment. I very rarely have such inspiration, but it felt right immediately. I wanted to have a silent "U" so BACUP stood for the British Association of Cancer Patients. Vicky felt strongly it should be the British Association of Cancer United Patients. This sounded to me like a football team, but for Vicky the concept of patients being united with each other and their family and friends, as well as their doctors, was important; so the name stuck.

About that time, Vicky was going on holiday to America and I introduced her to colleagues in a major cancer hospital in New York – The Memorial Sloan Kettering Hospital – and people in the National Cancer Institute in Bethesda, Maryland. Vicky came back, having met not only people to whom I introduced her, but many others. She spent an energetic few weeks in the United States, getting every bit of information she could about their cancer information services. She returned with suitcases full of information and practical ideas about how to set up BACUP. She dashed around the UK, meeting everybody who had anything to do with cancer services, every cancer doctor she could find and trying to convince them about the value of her idea. Once again, she managed to bring almost everyone with her. My anxiety about rejection by the medical profession did not materialise. Vicky acted as a bridge for conventional cancer doctors, who would not associate with alternative medicine, but wanted to find the best way to support their patients. Once again, her position as patient and doctor and her newly discovered charismatic personality, paid off. She spoke to senior doctors who previously might have intimidated her. She did not beg anyone for support; she won them over by her professional approach and inspiring personality. She was enthralled and energised by her reception. She regarded the new power and freedom cancer had given her as a child regards a new toy. She was starting to realise she had the freedom to break all the rules and initiate change herself. This was especially exciting for someone who had come from a hierarchical Eurasian family, where the women did not have much power.

Of course, part of the energy, enthusiasm and hurry to get things done was based on the knowledge she may relapse and her time be limited. If you are going to change the world and you might die of cancer, you cannot afford to waste time. Although Vicky was an extreme example of the altruism which often comes after a crisis, many patients experience similar desires. People with cancer who only had ambitions of a personal nature frequently find they have a much broader aim to life and a great need to contribute to others. This change in perspective towards a greater social involvement coming out of the cancer crisis is something that surprises many people, not least the family of a person with cancer. The family suddenly finds dinner being made on time is no longer a priority and bigger causes take precedence. These changes are not always welcomed by those closest to the cancer patient.

Perhaps it wasn't necessary to convince as many people as Vicky saw, but one of the major problems of starting something like BACUP is it can easily be seen as weird and possibly dangerous, or as amateurish and second-rate by the medical profession. Cancer doctors are conservative about what they are prepared to support and, as we know, the great majority of cancer patients are treated by conventional doctors. We felt it was important BACUP was seen as a highly professional organisation supported by the medical establishment, if it was going to succeed. There were a number of medical specialists who were crucial to establishing BACUP's role. Some of these were Professor Tim McElwain, Professor of Medicine at the Royal Marsden Hospital, Professor Kenneth Calman, Professor of Oncology at Glasgow and Dr Peter Wrigley, a medical oncologist at Bart's. These people enabled us to claim BACUP had the support of the medical establishment. They were convinced by Vicky to go out on a limb and risk some of their own credibility to help get BACUP established. In October 1984, 50 people met at a working party to give birth to the organisation. A steering committee was set up with Vicky as chairperson. This was the first committee Vicky had ever attended or chaired. She tackled the project, like all her others, with hours of preparation and thought. Every conclusion was planned and nothing was left to chance. Although the working party voted on who should comprise the steering committee and who should be officers of the organisation, Vicky had organised the nomination and seconding before the meeting. She also organised who should speak in support of each person. As a result of this entirely non-random process, I became deputy chairman, and Tim McElwain became chairman of the Medical Specialist Advisory Board. It is interesting, looking back, how we all accepted being organised by Vicky, without complaint and with a smile! It was because what she was doing was subtle and difficult to pick up, despite the fact that all of us had considerably more experience of committees and organisations than she did. Vicky had undergone a revolution. She was a leader and accepted as such by senior members of the medical, nursing and related professions.

When Vicky first asked me to join her in setting up BACUP, I wondered whether getting involved was a good idea. Despite our friendship, I was concerned that working together might make it more difficult to maintain the essential relationship as her doctor. I was conscious of the fact she had a very good chance of relapsing. She convinced me she very much wanted me to join her in this and she needed my help to get it off the ground. She wanted me to be her deputy, as I had, in practice, been involved with the project right from the very beginning. I thought once again this was an unusual situation, she had a very good idea and I should break with convention and ignore the standard rules. I agreed to work with her despite the fact she was my patient. We ended up with not two, but three different roles. There was the role as her friend based on equality, the doctor/patient relationship where the doctor has the stereotyped superior role, and with BACUP, where she was the boss. My relationship with Vicky became very interesting because we engaged in this conscious form of role play. We had decided, as I mentioned earlier, that there was a time for the doctor/patient relationship when she was the patient and the doctor has the authority, then if we talked about BACUP, we switched roles again. When we were relating as friends, we changed position again. So essentially what we were doing was switching authorities.

I think this role play was very important to avoid confusion and conflict which could have arisen from mixing roles in this way. Clearly our relationship was based on mutual respect and affection, and a common enthusiasm for her project. There was no doubt we were able to stimulate each other's ideas and could always work extremely enjoyably and comfortably together. I think my colleagues always regarded our relationship and the seemingly confusing roles with amusement and some degree of puzzlement. Certainly everyone in the Medical Oncology Department knew we were friends as well as colleagues, and this made the junior doctors somewhat nervous when they were treating her. Some of my colleagues commented they did not think the potentially conflicting roles were suitable. I simply agreed it was essentially problematic, but there were times when one had to ignore the rules. I felt it would be a pity if we were so hidebound by rules they could never be altered.

*Vicky:* Maurice and I were a partnership. I used to look forward to him coming to visit me. When he told me I may be cured after 14 months of treatment I felt a great sense of loss at the cord being cut. The cord being between myself and the hospital and between myself and Maurice. There was, of course, a time when I became very depressed and had a big dip in my life. I am a doctor and so I know all about the doctor/patient relationship and its importance. Maurice talked to me about my illness, my symptoms and examined me. I wanted to talk to him about my worries and depressions and he listened. We were also great friends and a good partnership. Maurice had a difficult time in relation to his family and got divorced. I was upset with him because I was one of the last ones to be told. He explained it was a way of protecting me because I had too much on my plate. But I was angry he had done that because we were a team and I realised the relationship wasn't equal. He was supporting me and didn't allow me to give him support when he was having difficulties.

*Maurice:* BACUP was a new dimension for me. Over the past year I had been involved in setting up support groups and doing counselling courses. BACUP offered me the opportunity to become involved in trying to provide a better support for cancer patients throughout the country. Everyone who was involved felt this was something special. There was a feeling of "togetherness", of creating something new, almost a pioneer spirit inspired by the need and by Vicky's enthusiasm. Just a few months before, no-one had thought of a cancer information service. Now we were convinced we could not do without one. Getting senior members of the medical profession to support the start of an organisation is very difficult. To get them to attend meetings regularly on top of other commitments is virtually impossible; yet they came every time to the steering committee meetings. Professor Calman flew down from Glasgow, Professor McElwain came up from Sutton. They were caught up in the feeling this was something worthwhile. So we met regularly and planned for the launch of BACUP, with Vicky continuing to chair and, in fact, direct the meetings in her own inimitable style.

Initially Vicky planned to set up BACUP while running her general practice. When she became ill again she decided to work with BACUP full-time. BACUP looked as though it was going to be bigger than we had originally anticipated. It would have been unrealistic for her to do this at the same time as setting up general practice, especially as she now required more treatment. It became apparent BACUP needed a lot more than we had initially thought. First, it needed money. It is one thing applying for grants when you are actually established; it is another trying to get going when you are nothing more than an idea. You do not have an office, you are not providing a service and people are very unlikely to give you money before you are a reality. Vicky managed to raise money first by twisting the arms of her relatives, particularly her father. Substantial sums were also donated by individual patients and relatives. We ended up with nearly £80,000. We were given an office by Bart's Trustees, rent free for one year. So BACUP was founded by a few enthusiastic individuals prepared to take a big risk because the idea grabbed them and they were enthralled with Vicky. Everybody knows charities come and go; they start with enthusiasm, and quickly fail.

*Vicky:* When I was a doctor I was doing research into endocrinology on natural morphines and acupuncture. I was working in the laboratory looking after patients on the ward with hormone problems. I was never my own boss. I worked for very powerful professors. I had never done anything like BACUP before; I never started something which is entirely mine, with me in charge. It feels great, a lot better than working for someone else, because when you are working for yourself at something you really want to do, it just feels right. When you are working for other people, you are sometimes working for the wrong motives, for example, working to please people who you may need to qualify or to prove something. BACUP is something I really believe in and it has become the most important thing in my life since I first thought about it.

## THE NEED TO LIVE

*Maurice:* Just before the first steering committee meeting, Vicky relapsed. This was terribly disappointing for me as well as for her. She was no longer just another patient and I felt a degree of personal responsibility. Although I was satisfied she had received the correct treatment, I could not help feeling I had failed her. Vicky faced the situation in exactly the same way as the initial illness, but there was less panic and less activity. She had experienced this before, so it was not all unknown. Once again, we went back to providing information about everything available. We talked to Tim and David, and with her family. Vicky was depressed for only a short time. The formation of BACUP gave her a project on which to concentrate and help lift her depression. Many people might argue a sick person shouldn't work so hard. They should rest and conserve their energy. For Vicky, and many other patients in a similar situation, becoming involved in a meaningful project has the opposite effect. It gives energy and helps combat depression.

Vicky had to have another major operation and had her rectum removed. She had a colostomy, "a bag". She understood now it was unlikely she would be cured. In fact she had a way of talking to people about that, she used to say, "If I get run over by a bus I want to make sure that BACUP is OK." She didn't want to embarrass people by saying, "If I die from cancer ...." She was once or twice asked by journalists, "What do you think is going to happen to you?" "How long do you think you are going to live?" She answered by saying, "If you are asking me whether I think I will collect my old age pension, I guess that is unlikely." It seemed to me her attitude to her prognosis was a very healthy and successful way of dealing with an impossible situation. She told me it was very important for her to be alive at the launch of BACUP in October 1985. Vicky set herself relatively short-term goals that were attainable and when she achieved them she had a feeling of satisfaction. The disease got worse. This was now a very difficult situation and it was clear standard therapy was not going to work. We needed to find a new approach with a chance of overcoming the seemingly impossible. I phoned a colleague at another hospital who was trying a very new treatment using high doses of chemotherapy and bone marrow transplantation. The effect of this was unknown. In theory it was the only chance of tackling Vicky's disease. Vicky, of course, knew all this, but would rather try a new treatment with even a very slight chance of working, than accept that very little could be done. From my own point of view, I was relieved at being able to share the burden of her care with a colleague. It was a great support to me and from then on I used to discuss treatment decisions with him. This was particularly valuable at a later stage when decisions became even more difficult. Being a consultant is very lonely at times. You always can and do discuss patients with colleagues, but the final responsibility and decision rest with you. Actually having somebody else whom I respected involved with Vicky's treatment made it much easier for me, especially as I was now treating a close friend. Colleagues sometimes suggested I refer Vicky to someone else, as I may not have been able to make rational decisions in view of our friendship. I have no doubt this would have been a mistake. Vicky would have seen it as me abandoning her when she most needed support. So the opportunity to share her care with a colleague was a great bonus for me.

Vicky had the high-dose chemotherapy treatment. She responded quite well with partial remission of the cancer, felt better and returned to work full-time at BACUP. About 9 months later she relapsed again. I treated her with a new drug being used in ovarian cancer, but this did not help at all and the disease grew further. By now she had very advanced disease. Her bowels were blocked with cancer and she couldn't eat. Both kidneys were also blocked, so she was going into kidney failure and she also had pneumonia. She was obviously extremely ill. Her abdomen was bloated because of the blocked bowels, and she needed a tube through her nose into her stomach to stop her vomiting continuously. The blocked kidneys resulted in waste products accumulating in her blood, causing her to feel sick. She was short of breath and needed oxygen because of the pneumonia. At this point I spoke to her and Tim about whether it was really worthwhile treating her pneumonia, kidney failure and blocked bowels. I looked at Vicky lying in bed, with advanced ovarian cancer, that had now grown despite all standard and some experimental treatment. I felt extremely sad and desperate for her. I knew how much she wanted to live, but I also knew if she were to live, it would be a very difficult time from here on. I asked myself the question, "Would I want to live in this situation?" The answer was a clear, "no". I asked myself what would I advise my mother or sister to do in this situation. I felt I had to tell Vicky and Tim what I thought. It was very difficult for me.

It was not unusual for me to have to talk to a patient in this way, but with Vicky it felt different. I felt personally responsible for her. She had so much faith in me and I had let her down. Although she was very ill she could think clearly and I spoke to her and Tim at the same time. I told her she would not benefit from any further chemotherapy at this point. The only possible treatment was hormonal therapy, but this had only a small chance of working and, in any event, its effectiveness would only be temporary. Even if she responded, in a short time she would have to face up to all these problems again. I felt we should consider not treating her pneumonia, as the kindest, gentlest thing to do for Vicky at this time was to let her die quietly in a respectful, dignified way. She understood very clearly I was suggesting we did not give her any more active treatment, but make her feel comfortable and let her die. It is the only time in our relationship she became angry with me. She said to me calmly and very coldly, there was no possibility of her accepting that. She wanted more information about the hormonal treatment.

Hormones are occasionally helpful in ovarian cancer and can even temporarily shrink the cancer in a small minority of patients. These cannot "cure" the patient and for most patients do not help at all. I told her these details and said I would be happy to give the treatment if that was what she wanted. The problem was, because of her blocked bowels, she had to be fed continually by a drip into a vein. She would also need to have a tube in her back to drain her blocked kidneys and, if her bowels continued to be blocked, she might have to consider a tube to drain her stomach; a gastrostomy. Both she and Tim, without even discussing it, told me politely and calmly that was what they wanted, so could I please organise it? I knew I had completely misjudged the situation and there was no way Vicky would be prepared to give up. I felt awful at the time I had caused her so much distress, but I could not have carried on without confirmation this was what she really wanted.

## DIFFICULT DECISIONS : WHO MAKES THEM?

*Maurice:* It is very difficult for a doctor to decide at what point to stop treatment. It is common for cancer doctors to have to talk to people about these issues and make these decisions. Who says doctors can or should make these decisions? It is clearly a big burden society places on doctors and at many times you have to go on nothing other than intuition. I believe the only people who can ultimately make these decisions are the patient and family. The doctor can and does consider what he or she would want personally for his or her own family, but this is not necessarily right for everyone. The difficulty is how to give the patient the opportunity to make their own decision without creating distress, by discussing the issue in the first place. But I still felt that I had let Vicky down. I was someone who was supposed to know her well and be her good friend. I felt I should have guessed she would not accept the idea of no treatment. However, during the following year, I was very glad I had that discussion. There were times when some colleagues felt my treatment of Vicky was inappropriately aggressive. At these times the knowledge I was doing what she wanted was very helpful. Despite this, some colleagues felt I was being manipulated by Vicky and I should simply make the decision to stop treatment. At times I, too, wondered if this was not "modern medicine gone mad".

Vicky then started to organise and get busy. First, her family flew in from Australia, New York, Los Angeles, Hong Kong and all over the world. I felt fairly sure she was going to die despite the hormone treatment. Vicky telephoned every member of the BACUP steering committee on her portable phone and said, "Listen, things are not looking very good, I am quite ill." Even at this stage she did not want sympathy. BACUP had now been launched for 3 or 4 months and she asked the executives to agree to Tim becoming a trustee of the charity. Up to that point Tim had not been involved, except in the background supporting and guiding her. Vicky hated "Mum and Dad charities", charities set up as family affairs. She felt this interfered with professionalism. But when she thought she was dying she wanted to make sure her husband was there to ensure the charity was kept on the "straight and narrow", in other words, she was trying to make sure her wishes were carried out after she died.

Vicky's decision went against my own feelings about what life is about. For me life with tumours all over the body, being fed by a drip, together with discomfort and pain, was not worth living. Vicky was not asking my opinion about what I thought about life. She made her own decisions. She just asked for my skills to help her to achieve what she needed. She considered the options, made her decisions and never looked back. It was clear Vicky and I thought differently. She wanted to live, almost at any cost. She once said to me, "You can do anything you like below the neck. I don't care what you do to my body, provided my mind is OK." It wasn't the fact she didn't care about her body, she cared very much. She was a physical person who enjoyed every aspect of life, including food, sport and sex, but to live was more important than anything else. I followed her wishes. I treated her pneumonia, put in a drip to feed her and asked a surgical colleague to put in a tube to drain her kidneys. I also started giving her the hormonal treatment.

Vicky remained angry with me for weeks. She did not express this directly, but her friendly enthusiasm was replaced by cold distance. She was also irritated with the nurses and doctors on the ward for the first time in her illness. I am sure the anger was not directed simply at me and, to a degree, was anger at the situation in which she found herself. Anger is an important component of coming to terms with illness and change for many people. What is surprising is how little anger she had felt or expressed before.

## SURVIVING ON DRIVE ALONE

*Maurice:* Vicky went home understanding this was probably the end of her life. She organised a nurse to look after her, her GP to come in and see her frequently and a team from the local hospice to look after pain control. Of course, I also visited her regularly at home. Amazingly, dying became another project. She talked about writing an article, "Life after terminal care diagnosis", and I had no doubt she would have, had she felt well enough. However, all her careful preparations for terminal care were wasted. Not only did she respond to the hormonal treatment, she responded dramatically. The cancer shrank to about one-third its previous size. The tube going into her kidneys was removed, because her kidneys started working again. Unfortunately, her bowels did not start working properly and eventually it was necessary to put a tube into her stomach to drain its contents. She loved eating and all this time had been unable to eat. She developed a technique which she called "chewing and spitting". It is the first time I have ever heard of anyone doing it. She went out for gourmet meals at restaurants and she ate, enjoyed the food, chewed it, and then discreetly removed it from her mouth. She said you can actually train yourself to do that and enjoy food almost as much as swallowing it. Once again, it was another challenge successfully met.

She still had a lot of cancer and was walking around with tubes coming from everywhere and had to feed herself every night by connecting herself to a drip. Despite all this, she carried on with television appearances, working at BACUP, going in at least 1 or 2 days most weeks. She was in and out of hospital; one crisis after another; infections, illness, admitted to intensive care, close to death and rescued again. Despite all this she lived life and enjoyed it. She went to the Chelsea Flower Show and on holiday to Jersey for 2 weeks. It required a mammoth operation with her drip feeding being airlifted to Jersey. She went to Hong Kong for 2 weeks. Once again crates of drip feeding had to be airlifted and the Hilton Hotel had to buy a new refrigerator to cope with it. In Hong Kong Vicky was interviewed and appeared in a major article in the *South China Times*. Her origins were in Hong Kong. It was very important for her to go back as a success and having clearly made a major contribution. She took a nurse with her, in order to be looked after while she was there and enjoyed herself enormously. She took more pleasure from every moment of life when she was not feeling ill than most people would in a month or even a year.

*Vicky:* I enjoy life. Tim always says that you only need to give me a little pleasure, a treat in terms of what I can do in relation to my illness, and I am happy. Going to a restaurant for the first time, or being pushed around in a wheelchair at a horticultural gardens, or going to Wimbledon against all the odds. Sometimes I think of myself as a hedonist and I just enjoy life too much. Tim, David and me do many things together; play the piano, go places. We are all great friends, a trio as such.

*Maurice:* Looking back, it is a sobering thought that I had suggested 18 months previously that Vicky stop treatment. These months might well have been the most important months of her life. At the time I suggested it to her it felt the right decision. Yet, over those 18 months she did so much to get the charity off the ground, to publicise it and win over the hearts and minds of many people. BACUP became the centre of her life. She was surrounded by friends and family and BACUP. She was obsessed with BACUP and made a unique contribution, especially with the newspapers and on television programmes. Anyone she met could not fail to be impressed by her. She was clearly very ill and yet had this energy and enthusiasm. She dragged herself out of her hospital bed to appear on the Wogan chat show. She went on another television programme which lasted from 12 midnight to 3 a.m. She maintained a feeling of hope right until the very end.

Vicky died on Thursday and on the Friday afternoon before that, 6 days before she died, she was planning a holiday to the lakes of northern Italy. I had organised with the Home Office for her to take her morphine out of the country so she could inject herself in Italy. She was really looking forward to that holiday. On one level she accepted the fact she was going to die and, on another, she was completely unrealistic. Two weeks before she died we had a discussion which illustrated this point. I had a special tube manufactured for her gastrostomy, the tube into her stomach. It was quite an effort to get the company to reset the machines, but eventually they made two dozen tubes. Two weeks before she died Vicky asked me how many tubes I had left and I told her we had 24. She reminded me it took 6 months to have them made and asked that I planned in advance so there was no delay next time. She calculated as each lasted about 3 months, 24 would last about 6 years. She asked me to please reorder at least 1 year in advance, that is in 5 years' time, so she did not run out of tubes.

Despite this she was very clear about what was happening. She existed on the one hand with this feeling of total reality and, on the other hand, and at the same moment, she could talk completely unrealistically about how long she expected to live. I think, actually, this is a good example of how many people behave. It is uncommon for people, excepting when they are very close to death, to really come to terms with dying. People seem to co-exist easily with two completely conflicting thoughts. Vicky was totally absorbed in what she was doing. She demonstrated how you could have maximum information and still selectively deny what you do not want to think about. Some people, even doctors and nurses, found her approach irritating. They could not understand why she did not die in peace. There was never an aura of sadness or depression or pity around Vicky. Anyone who talked to her knew she was living every moment to the full.

## ONGOING INSPIRATION

*Maurice:* Her death was very peaceful. She slipped quietly into drowsiness and then unconsciousness. The day she died she was surrounded by her husband and close friends, David, Alison and Michael, by myself and Yvonne from BACUP. People from the hospital and all over London popped in just to wave "goodbye", even though Vicky could not consciously appreciate their presence. As with her life, it was not a depressing time; that came later. There was a feeling of elation, a paradoxical "high", we all experienced as we stood and talked and joked about Vicky. To some this might sound disrespectful, cynical or even sick. It was not planned, it just happened. It was appropriate, it just felt right to everyone.

Looking back it is clear Vicky influenced me enormously. I often hear patients say how they are influenced by their doctor, but it is less common for a doctor to be very influenced by a patient. I met Vicky shortly after taking up a consultant post. I was interested in communication and support groups. Vicky provided me with a private course in communication with cancer patients. If anything I said did not make sense or was confusing, she told me so. She had the ability to criticise without offending, and constantly taught me what she needed, simply by demanding it. Much of Vicky's behaviour was extreme, but she used the same coping mechanisms many other people find very helpful. An intuitive understanding of the enormous emotional benefit of information, setting small goals and rearranging priorities, is helpful to anyone dealing with a crisis in life, not just cancer. She made me think about patients and doctors as partners or colleagues in dealing with an illness, and I have never seen the doctor/patient relationship in the same light since. She showed me how important it is for people to be involved in decisions about their own lives and that doctors cannot accurately project their own feelings onto their patients.

I was very fortunate to meet Vicky at such an early stage in my career because she made me aware of many things which now affect the way I relate to all my patients. She understood and practised Nira Kfir's model of crisis intervention without needing to be taught. In fact, the model is a description of successful coping behaviour in times of crisis and enables us to intervene appropriately/helpfully when people are not dealing with the crisis successfully. Vicky taught others by example how to cope with illness and even death. Through BACUP she enabled many people who never met her, and others who have never heard of her, to benefit from her insight, her enthusiasm and, most of all, her inspiration.

## UNDERSTANDING VICKY

*Maurice:* I have always had a need to understand. I asked Nira to talk to Vicky because I was baffled by how Vicky found her courage, her ability to suffer with no self-pity and how new leadership qualities emerged in her after she developed cancer. I have always felt, since some people use better ways of coping than others, it should be possible to learn and reproduce these coping strategies, and other people could benefit from understanding Vicky's motives and conduct. In a simplistic way, I wanted to know what could be learnt and taught from Vicky's story.

*Nira:* We can learn from Vicky's story in the same way we can learn from *Alice in Wonderland*, *Gone with the Wind*, the *Bible* or *Dynasty*. To use Bernie Siegal's words, "It cannot be taught, it can only be learned." It is not the example that is learned – no more than we learn from Hannibal's bravery, Napoleon's victories or Mother Teresa's devotion. It is a certain part of the story that fits our own understanding of life and sets a spark in us, that makes it possible for us too.

Many times I have heard people say, "This movie changed my life", or, "Did you read that novel, it transformed me." Whenever I took the time to go and see this transforming movie I was strongly disappointed. Yet it did inspire someone; it created movement and change. The whole of therapy is telling and sharing stories. The rest, the real therapy, happens in between the stories.

We know already crisis and change are not triggered by the events themselves, but by our interpretation of them. Adler's *Psychology of Human Nature* teaches us that a child, in the formative years, builds his or her own personality, not so much because of what happens, but by his or her interpretation of those events (Adler 1957). It is this which forms a unique personality and lifestyle. The child is a sharp observer, but a rather limited interpreter. This only means that, even as young as 3 years old, we find it hard to just exist, without having a personal philosophy of life. So we create one. The materials used are family, events, experience and observations. The child, once he or she has assumed what life is, uses experiences to confirm his or her own assumptions.

*Maurice:* Can we determine Vicky's personal philosophy of life from her story about herself?

*Nira:* When I spoke to Vicky she told me about her childhood and early memories. Alfred Adler showed these early memories tell a lot about how a person views life. It is not the memories themselves, but the fact a person remembers them that is significant. This book is not about psychology, but I think understanding the way Vicky saw life will help us to understand how she behaved when she developed cancer.

This is how Vicky told her life story.

**ON HER OWN LIFE**

*Vicky:* I was born in Hong Kong, the third of five children. My father is Chinese from Indonesia and my mother comes from a very old Eurasian (mixed Chinese and European) family in Hong Kong. The original English/Dutch traders who went to Hong Kong took Chinese wives, and those mixed marriages produced children between the Chinese and European community, who had a very important function. They belonged to the Chinese community, yet were different because they had European blood. This gave them considerable influence and they liaised between traders and the Chinese community. My mother's family is very famous in Hong Kong, and my great uncle was knighted. They were wealthy and influential. My father's family were not very successful. My father's father was a customs officer in Indonesia, nothing very grand. My father has been manic all his life. I don't mean manic in the pathological sense, but he has always had a hyperactive personality, which makes him very difficult to live with. My mother had great difficulty managing. They had five children, and when the youngest was 4 years old, she decided, even though she had a large extended family in Hong Kong, she would leave my father and go to live in England. There is still a strong bond between my mother and father, even though they have been separated for many years. My father always supported us financially. He was a successful business man, and wealthy enough to do this.

My role in the family was very difficult. My perception as a child was that I was unwanted. Chinese families don't value girls; there is an expression for daughters, which is "spare baggage". I wasn't the eldest or the youngest, I was the one in the middle, the "sandwich squeeze" child. My younger brother, Ronnie, was the favourite, because he was born at a time of good fortune. We were living in Burma at the time and my father's business was starting to go well. He doted on his youngest son. My father is very superstitious. I had been born at a time when he was down on his luck and he blamed me. When I was born we were living in a slum tenement. I used to have colic when I was a baby and cry frequently, keeping them awake. He tells a story about putting me in the bathroom and threatening to flush me down the loo. This is meant to be a funny story when he tells it, but it really upsets me.

We were brought up by an amah, a servant who looks after children. The amah adored the boys. My elder sister had a lot of attention lavished on her because she was the first child; my younger sister demanded attention by being bad tempered. I didn't seem to have any tools to get my own way and I remember thinking it was very unfair. If we had to choose sweets, we either started with the eldest choosing first and going down, or the youngest choosing first and going up. I was always in the middle and I never chose first.

**EARLY RECOLLECTIONS**

*Vicky:* Something else that sticks in my mind happened in Burma. My elder brother fell over and was cut over his eye. I was blamed for it because I had left the paper he tripped over on the floor. I will never forget that. I can still see the verandah where he tripped, the scar he had afterwards. I remember when I was about 6, we were all playing tambourines, xylophones and drums. We were squabbling about who was to play what. My father was angry and stood us in a row. Not the youngest, because they were too small, just my elder sister, my brother and me. We were very well-behaved children; we didn't usually make any noise because we were so petrified of him. He stood us in a row and made us slap ourselves, telling us to do it harder and harder and harder.

When I was about 7, I was given a doctor's set. My father said we want a lawyer in the family and a doctor. I was given the doctor's set, and that is why I became a doctor. Well, I suppose not just because of that. I used to like helping people, and I dreamed about how I would invent a machine to put on people's tummies, which would convey to me how they felt and where the pain was exactly, so I would be able to help them. This machine was magic, because I would know where the pain was and would be able to make it go away. Another dream I had when I was a very young child was about an aeroplane crashing in the field. These were the fields opposite where we lived and I would go to the fields, to the aeroplane, and would be the heroine. I would save the people. I would be incredible.

We came to England by boat and sailed for months. I was on a boat for the first time, met many people and it was very exciting. I remember meeting a Japanese man, who made me realise I was quite a special child. In England we lived in East Grinstead, the five of us, my mother and the amah. There were no Chinese families in East Grinstead and a lot of racial prejudice. My mother was very attractive, people were very frightened she would take their husbands. We actually had no friends for many years, except widows.

## IMMIGRATION: CHANGE OF LUCK

*Vicky:* Coming to England did me a lot of good. I found out I was intelligent and could get attention by excelling. I thought I would do well at school and if I worked hard, I would find my own niche. I tried to excel at everything. I was a very good pianist; the best pianist in the school. I took all the exams and passed with distinctions. I was also a sportsperson and captain of all the teams. I also played for county hockey. My achievements gave me great pleasure. My brother went to Cambridge and I thought, "Gosh, wouldn't it be fantastic, even though I went to a school which never sent people to Cambridge?" I was determined to go and, when I took the exams and didn't get in, I was very disappointed. I decided to try again and got in the second time. I graduated with a double first, which was better than my brother.

Cambridge gave me something else. Right at the beginning I met my husband to be, Tim, and we have been together ever since. Being with him has completely shaped my life. He really gave me the reason to be alive and gave me something of my own. Having him as a boyfriend was something of mine my family couldn't take away. It was something I had chosen. I had chosen to leave East Grinstead, go to university and make a new life. Tim is a lawyer. I have been very lucky with him. We really were friends as well as boyfriend and girlfriend. I always thought I didn't want to marry someone from the same sort of dormitory town I came from. Tim, however, lived only 20 minutes away, yet had the same horizons to which I aspired. He was also one of five and a middle child. So I left home and immediately made another bond. Looking back, I have never really been on my own. I also met my best friend, Alison, at Cambridge and we have been best friends ever since. I am not very gregarious. I don't make a lot of friends, but my relationships are longstanding. I have another very close friend, who is also a close friend of Tim's, David. David is a GP, but was my registrar when I did my first job as house officer in hospital, after I qualified in 1973. I talk to him most days. Some husbands would be jealous, but Tim is not and the three of us have a wonderful friendship. I am really very lucky.

About 3 three years after qualifying, I started working at St Bartholomew's Hospital for incredibly dynamic, powerful professors, who were world famous. I was a junior doctor and was offered a research job. It was an offer I couldn't refuse. I threw myself into research and decided I was going to "lick it". At the time, natural morphines had just been discovered. I had no scientific experience but, within a year and a half, I developed a new method to measure a new natural morphine. It was published in major medical journals. I worked extremely hard, pushing myself to the limit. Thinking back, it was probably to please my professors, similar to trying to please my father. It was also something I did for myself, to prove I could do it.

## OBSERVATIONS

*Maurice:* I have known Vicky since she was diagnosed and have heard her life story from her and bits and pieces from her family. Talking to Vicky and observing her would not have led me to picture her in the way she presents herself here. This powerful, optimistic person seemed to start her life with a rather fatalistic and pessimistic philosophy of what life was about.

   *Nira:* Everything in Vicky's childhood pointed, in her view, to a total lack of control over life. She was born at a time when her father was "down on his luck". So in a way she was part of it. Luck, of course, is not negotiable, whether or not one accepts it. Another thing she had to accept was she was born a girl. This, too, is bad luck, since girls are "spare baggage". By the time Vicky tried to come to terms with these "great disadvantages", she discovered it is not only luck, but also people who cannot be changed. The people in her family, from her father down, were perceived as remote. Father personified to Vicky the frightening and unexpected. Not to mean anything to him made her meaningless. Fear, unfairness and impotence were her basic conceptions of life.

   What was life to Vicky? Looking at her early memories, one can build a picture. Life was dangerous and survival was doubtful. "You were flushed down the toilet", next time you may really go down. Can you control father's anger? Can you understand the logic of your punishment? There was none. She was punished personally because her brother slipped on a piece of paper. She was punished collectively for unknown reasons. One reality seems to be persistent – pain. Neither the pain nor the colic annoyed her father, just her incessant crying. She learned that letting the world know about her pain was worse than the pain itself. She also learned one cannot control life, one cannot even control the pain in one's own body.

   In a later memory, we can really see the formation of a solution. When the children stand in line and have to slap themselves, Vicky is not crying any more. Vicky slaps herself harder and harder in a moment that may seem like total surrender, but is not. Vicky formed in those first years, between the toilet episode and the "collective punishment", her own priority and greatest asset, self-control. She stands there hitting herself, pain without complaint, unseen pain, meaningless pain, denied pain. The denial of pain means control. The pain itself cannot be controlled, but at least she can control her response.

*Maurice:* Her attitude towards pain control was amazing. Vicky carried on as if pain, not to mention physical inconvenience, didn't count. Her almost total absence of complaint made one often forget how "inconvenient" it must be to live with bags, spit out food and be a living mechanism.

*Nira:* Not every child sees lack of control as a major issue in life. Millions of other Chinese girls, and of course others, grow up in the same milieu, but each one chooses to focus on a different aspect of life. Vicky observed and assessed life as being uncontrollable. In her personal struggle for control she was equipped with only one asset – herself – her body, her willpower and her mind. In her young adulthood in England, we listen to Vicky using these assets. She excels in almost everything she does: school, sports, piano. We can see the control went much higher than just survival. Vicky tried to conquer nearly every field in which she became interested. Hard work, overcoming failures and trying again were the means.

*Maurice:* Are you suggesting overcoming a person's greatest fear becomes their major goal? Since Vicky pictured life as uncontrollable, and therefore dangerous, she made control her number one priority?

*Nira:* For Vicky, loss of control was an impasse. Being in control became a priority to be repeated and regained in every new field. Apart from control, another major goal in her life was the search for meaning. The goal of control is survival and the means of achieving control are self-discipline, self-manipulation, self-sufficiency, self-extension and autonomy. Meaning is something you cannot give yourself. Meaning is given to a person at any age by another person or people. No matter how self-sufficient you are, you cannot give yourself meaning. Vicky speaks about being "unloved and meaningless" in the eyes of her family. Not only her father, but also the amah, ignored her and didn't love her.

Being loved and cared for in early life makes us feel we have a right to survive. Being rejected makes us doubt our basic right to exist and take up space in this world. Vicky never took her place for granted. She believed she had to justify her life, her "pot luck" entry into the world, by contributions. She decided that, even if she didn't mean much to her family, she would still become unique. Her dreams represent her ideal of what her life should be and how indispensable she may become.

In the fantasy of the plane crash in the field near her house people are crushed, again one of life's inevitable catastrophes, and she, only she, runs to the rescue. She dreams of becoming a heroine. To be in the right place at the right time, to save and rescue others. In another memory, given a medical kit to play with, Vicky dreams of inventing a pain detector which will show where pain is, and how to make the pain go away.

*Maurice:* I have often thought of heroism when talking to people close to death. The doctor can only help with pain control and general minimising of suffering. The acceptance of the situation, by the patient, always struck me as heroic. It is not overcoming death, it is struggling with the fear of death that never fails to surprise me. Vicky, more than anyone else, seemed as if she not only won this battle, but that it didn't exist at all. Part of her specialness was rooted in her lack of fear of death.

*Nira:* Ernest Becker, a psychologist and author of *The Denial of Death*, describes what you call "lack of fear of death" (Becker 1973). He claims death and the fear of it are the greatest motivators of human behaviour. Life itself is denial of death, but since the fear of death is so overwhelming, we have to deny and repress not just death, but the fear of it. The fear of death is our threat, even more than death itself. Denial demands a great amount of energy which is spent, all through life, on just one cause, repressing the fear of death.

Since death is inherent in every life, we are actually denying not death itself, but the time and the way we die. These two are our only bargaining chips. But a diagnosis of cancer confronts us with the time and cause of our death, the two facts we don't want to know, and our ability to deny the fear of death is strongly challenged.

*Maurice:* Many people at that point do "more of the same". Even more energy is spent on the denial of the fear of death.

*Nira:* More of the same is one way of coping. It requires a great effort to go on with life, the way it was lived. For many people denial becomes so consuming no energy is left for life. Depression, general loss of vital energy, becomes life. Depression and repression seem still a better option than confronting the fear of death.

*Maurice:* Most people I have seen in this situation try to go on with life, including the denial of death, to the end. This denial is helpful to the doctor as well, as he or she can still communicate with the person and they have a common goal. The acceptance of death makes communication much more difficult.

*Nira:* While most people, confronted with reality of when and how, can still repress the fear of death, some people, a minority, are the exceptions. The defences of these individuals are hit by the bomb of confrontation. One cancer patient described it is this way:

I lived all my life as a city under siege. Life is going on in the city, but all depends on the thick wall protecting it, separating it from the enemy threatening to destroy it. The walls, by being strong and solid, guarantee life. But, if the walls collapse, the city is exposed and life cannot go on. Although the city may not have been touched, simply the collapse of the walls makes life impossible. There are only two ways left, to go on living as if more walls exist, hiding behind doors, under beds, or even behind curtains, or change direction and strike back.

This metaphor is part of the history of every nation. The time before war, being threatened, fear, anxiety, loss of hope, fear of death, can hardly be denied. Then comes the decision made by the leadership of the nation, to start war. The change is dramatic. People who yesterday were afraid and depressed now run towards yesterday's dangers as if they had disappeared. The vast national energy spent on fear and denial was released, the dam collapsed and the waters flood the land. The enormous energy creates a transformation, it turns fear into heroism.

Heroism, then, is the greatest denial of death itself. This transformation from paralysing fear to active fighting can occur only at the lowest point of despair. When there is "nothing to lose", why not "fall asleep and go"?

Cynical as our times are, we are still thrilled by a story about an unknown person who runs into a burning house to save a baby. So heroism can be transformed fear and it may not even be a conscious choice. Being afraid of death all one's life, then running into the flames, is called heroic, why not suicidal? It seems this dramatic change releases the forces spent on protecting our own survival to a new direction: survival of others.

*Maurice:* This is also true of Vicky. Initially her energies were directed towards saving her life. Only when the cancer relapsed and her greatest fear became uncontrollable did all this energy become available to her. She moved from focusing on the need to survive and preserve her own life to helping others.

*Nira:* The moment the fear of death disappears, a great power is released, as Becker (1973) describes it. Vicky became heroic, not in not wanting to live, but in her courage to live her dream. She became the heroine she dreamed of being; the one who saves people from a crashed plane, the one who tells people where the pain is and how they can be cured. The release of fear into action.

*Maurice:* Vicky changed her "pot luck" into success. Becker's description is actually her own, "Cancer freed me" (Becker 1973).

*Nira:* Aristotle described luck by saying "Luck is when the other man is hit by the arrow." Paraphrasing, we can say Vicky changed her luck when being the guy hit by the arrow. Can one, ill with cancer, be inspired by the story of Vicky Clement Jones? Can one overcome one's own fear of death by self-discovery? Vicky introduced us all to the idea of "cancer freedom". She used her own for the creation of a new cancer service; others may use it differently. The British media made Vicky a heroine, but those with her during her last years of life will realise heroism is the most natural thing for people, once they are free.

# References

Adler, A. (1957) *Understanding Human Nature*, (trans. W.B. Wolfe) Green-
wich, Conn.: Premier Books.
Adler, A. (1962) *What Life Should Mean to You*, London: Allen & Unwin.
Alex, M. and Alex, B. (1981) *Grandpa and Me*, Tring, Herts: Lion.
Becker, E. (1973) *The Denial of Death*, New York: Free Press.
Calman, K.C. (1984) 'Quality of life in cancer patients – an hypothesis', *Journal
of Medical Ethics* (10) 3: 124–7.
Corsini, R.J. (ed.) (1984) *Encyclopedia of Psychology*, New York: Wiley.
Frankl, V.E. (1959) *Man's Search for Meaning*, Washington: Washington
Square Press.
Harris, J. (1985) *The Value of Life*, London: Routledge & Kegan Paul.
Kfir, N. (1988) *Crisis Intervention Verbatim*, New York: Hemisphere.
Naisbitt, J. (1988) *Megatrends*, New York: Warner Books.
Siegal, B. (1989) *Love, Medicine and Miracles*, London: Arrow.
Varley, S. (1985) *Badger's Parting Gift*, Glasgow: Collins.
White, E.B. (1969) *Charlotte's Web*, London: Puffin.